Sickle-cell Disease

MEDICINE IN THE TROPICS SERIES

Already published

Tropical Venereology
O.P. Arya, A.O. Osoba and F.J. Bennett

Practical Epidemiology
Third edition
D.J.P. Barker with F.J. Bennett

Leprosy
Second edition
Anthony Bryceson and Roy E. Pfaltzgraff

Epidemiology and Community Health in Warm Climate Countries
Edited by Robert Cruikshank, Kenneth L. Standard and Hugh B.L. Russell

Methods in Neurological Examination
T.O. Dada

Diagnostic Pathways in Clinical Medicine
Second edition
B.J. Essex

Basic Eye Surgery
J.K. Galbraith

Poliomyelitis
R.L. Huckstep

Tuberculosis in Children
F.J.W. Miller

Eye Disease in the Tropics
F.C. Rodger

Paediatric Problems in Tropical Countries
Edited by M.J. Robinson and E.L. Lee

Sickle-cell Disease
A HANDBOOK FOR THE GENERAL CLINICIAN

Edited by
A.F. Fleming
on behalf of the Sickle-cell Club
of Nigeria

Foreword by

H. Lehmann
C.B.E., F.R.S.
Professor of Biochemistry
University of Cambridge

CHURCHILL LIVINGSTONE
EDINBURGH LONDON MELBOURNE AND NEW YORK 1982

CHURCHILL LIVINGSTONE
Medical Division of Longman Group Limited

Distributed in the United States of America by
Churchill Livingstone Inc., 19 West 44th Street, New
York, N.Y. 10036, and by associated companies,
branches and representatives throughout the world.

© Longman Group Limited 1982

All rights reserved. No part of this publication may be
reproduced, stored in a retrieval system, or transmitted
in any form or by any means, electronic, mechanical
photocopying, recording or otherwise, without the prior
permission of the publishers (Churchill Livingstone,
Robert Stevenson House, 1–3 Baxter's Place, Leith
Walk, Edinburgh, EH1 3AF).

First published 1982

ISBN 0 443 02037X

British Library Cataloguing in Publication Data
Sickle-cell disease. — (Medicine in the tropics series)
   1. Sickle cell anemia
   I. Fleming, A. F.   II. Series
   616.1'52   RC641.7.S5

Printed in Singapore by Selector Printing Co Pte Ltd

WH
170
S 566
1982

3 0001 00033 9871

83922

To Our Patients

The royalties from the sale of this Handbook will be paid to the Sickle-cell Club of Nigeria and will be devoted to the welfare of Nigerian children with sickle-cell disease.

Foreword

The interest in the sickling phenomenon arose outside Africa some 70 years ago. The people to whom it was a vital concern were, however, of African descent. It is true to say that there can hardly be an African south of the Sahara and north of the River Zambezi to whom 'sickling' and all that it involves is not of vital interest. Yet although there has been an intensive literature on sickle-cell anaemia and on sickle-cell trait in the continents of Europe and America, this present volume is the first of its kind written in Africa for Africans. Although primarily aimed at tropical Africa, it will be welcomed around the shores of the Mediterranean Sea, the Middle East and India, and indeed the Americas North and South, i.e. wherever sickle-cell disease confronts the medical profession, the public health administrator and the general public. The population movements since the Second World War have seen to it that few London Hospitals and doctors in the Midlands of England can remain aloof. Though numbers may not be large, immigrants from Greece and Italy have carried the gene to the antipodes.

Of the merits of this book are foremost the encompassing range it offers to the medical practitioner of the aspects of the disease itself, its genetics (so important for family advice), its history and its interplay with malaria, particularly in Africa, where it protects the young sickle-cell trait carrier against the deadly malignant tertian or falciparum malaria.

It is a short time in years but a long one in human endeavour that I was asking why sickle-cell anaemia, so well described in the United States, was not seen in Uganda. We now know that the affected infants died before they could develop the classical picture. With increasing treatment of infections and malnutrition the children are now growing up and surmounting the handicaps which used to weed out the hereditary anaemia before it developed. It is worth recalling that even in the United States there was a considerable interval of time between the description of sickle cells by Herrick in 1910 and the gradual realisation that sickle-cell anaemia is a

frequent disorder of public health interest. I have described elsewhere my visit to Herrick in 1954 when he told me that he did not
want to be remembered for the discovery of the 'bizarre' phenomenon of sickle cells but for his description of myocardial infarction. Similarly, the problem of sickle-cell disorders is now well
recognised in India, yet I recall that it was more than 40 years after
Herrick's discovery when Mary Cutbush (now Crookston) and I
went to India with the specific purpose to search for sickling there,
and it was only when the search was successful that the criticism of
this 'hair-brained' expedition came to an end.

This book is the first authoritative volume on sickle-cell disorders coming from Africa. It is profoundly gratifying that Dr
Fleming, the editor of this book, and his collaborators, all like him
members of medical faculties in Africa, have dedicated their royalties to the Sickle-Cell Club of Nigeria, a club of which they can
already be proud, just as I predict they will be proud of this present volume in years to come.

H. Lehmann

Preface

The authors agreed to write this book because so many patients are today receiving treatment and being given advice which they, the authors, think is inappropriate. The aim of this book is simply to provide the knowledge which is necessary to any doctor who has the care of patients with sickle-cell disease. As it has been estimated that in Nigeria alone, 30 000 children are born each year with sickle-cell disease, the need for a comprehensive text on the condition is apparent.

It is hoped that this book will be read by medical students preparing for their qualifying examinations and by doctors working in Africa or anywhere else in the world where the disease is encountered. Each chapter has been kept as short as possible and is followed by a list of suggested further reading; only for the historical introduction (Ch. 1) and the account of recent advances (Ch. 9) are there comprehensive lists of references.

The history of our knowledge of sickle-cell disease is discussed in the first chapter, both in oral traditions of Africa and in modern medicine since the original description by Herrick in 1910. The chapter continues with an account of the chemistry, function and inheritance of normal and abnormal haemoglobins in man, with emphasis on the peculiar nature of sickle haemoglobin (Hb-S). A true understanding of the clinical course of sickle-cell disease cannot be achieved unless the chemistry of this molecular disease is mastered.

The expression of these chemical abnormalities when Hb-S is inherited in the heterozygous state (sickle-cell trait) is the subject of Chapter 2. The high frequency of the sickle gene is due to the advantage enjoyed by sickle-cell trait carriers in areas where *Plasmodium falciparum* malaria is endemic. The nature and extent of this advantage are described, as are the extremely minor disadvantages which result from sickle-cell trait. The chapter closes with comments on the controversial subject of genetic counselling. The changes in the blood in sickle-cell disease and its laboratory diagnosis are the subjects of the third chapter; attention is focused on a handful only of laboratory tests, which are all that are required for the accurate diagnosis of sickle-cell disease.

The pathological effects of sickling on the blood and on the solid tissues of the body are discussed in Chapter 4 as an introduction to the three chapters covering the clinical manifestations and management of sickle-cell disease in childhood (Ch. 5), during and after puberty (Ch. 6), and during pregnancy (Ch. 7). These clinical chapters are complemented by an account of the radiological changes (Ch. 8).

Recent advances and some current research are described in the final chapter. Many claims are being made for treatment of sickle-cell disease, but at the time of writing, no specific treatment has been proved to be both safe and effective. A cautionary note is sounded which we hope will be heeded by any doctor who has some inspiration as to a cure for sickle-cell disease, or who is approached by others wishing to sell such a supposed cure. A beneficial and specific treatment will come sometime for certain, but it will not be ethically correct to administer it to all patients until its safety has been demonstrated and its effectiveness proved by carefully conducted trials. Until that day dawns, the authors hope that this text will be a guide to all who seek to ameliorate the course of sickle-cell disease in their patients.

1982   A.F.F.

Acknowledgements

We are grateful for permission to reproduce the following figures: Figure 1.1, Blackwell, Oxford; Figures 1.2 and 1.3, Thomas, Illinois, Figure 1.4, Academic Press, New York; Figure 1.5, Heinemann, London; Figure 1.7, Saunders, Pennsylvania; Figure 1.8, *New England Journal of Medicine*; Figure 1.9, US Department of Health, Education and Welfare, Bethesda.

Figures 2.1, 2.2, 2.3, 2.4, 2.5 and 3.1 were prepared by the Educational Aids Unit, Faculty of Medicine, Ahmadu Bello University, Zaria, and we thank Miss Abigail Fadugba for her skilled draughtsmanship. The photography of Figures 5.1, 5.2 and 5.3 and the preparation of Figures 8.5 and 8.6 were performed in the Medical Illustration Department, University College Hospital, Ibadan.

Finally, we thank Miss N. Onuegbu for her patience and accurate typing of the text in its final stages of preparation.

A.F.F.

Contributors

Ed. 'B. Attah, M.B., M.R.C. Path., F.N.M.C. Path, F.R.C.P. (C). Professor of Pathology, Ahmadu Bello University, Zaria, Nigeria

C.E. Effiong, M.B., M.R.C.P., D.C.H., F.W.A.C.P., F.M.C. Paed. Professor of Paediatrics, University of Calabar, Calabar, Nigeria; Secretary of the Sickle-Cell Club of Nigeria

G.J.F. Esan, Ph.D. Ibadan, M.B., F.R.C.P. Lond., F.M.C. Path. Nigeria, F.W.A.C.P. Professor of Haematology, University of Ibadan, Ibadan, Nigeria

E.M. Essien, M.D. Lond., F.M.C. Path. Nigeria, F.W.A.C.P. Professor of Haematology, University of Ibadan, Ibadan, Nigeria

A.F. Fleming, M.A., M.D. Cantab., F.R.C. Path., F.M.C. Path. Nigeria.
Professor of Haematology, Ahmadu Bello University, Zaria, Nigeria; President of the Sickle-Cell Club of Nigeria

K.A. Harrison, M.D. Lond., F.R.C.O.G., F.M.C.O.G. Nigeria. Professor of Obstetrics and Gynaecology, Port Harcourt University, Port Harcourt, Nigeria

H.H.M. Knox-Macaulay, M.A., M.D. Cantab., M.R.C.P. Lond., F.R.C.P. Edin., F.W.A.C.P., D.T.M. and H. Professor of Haematology, Ahmadu Bello University, Zaria, Nigeria

S.B. Lagundoye, M.B., B.S. Lond., D.M.R.D. Edin., F.M.C.R. Nigeria, F.W.A.C.S.
Professor of Radiology, University of Ibadan, Ibadan, Nigeria

Contents

Definitions and abbreviations

Sickle-cell trait (Hb-AS): the inheritance of one normal gene controlling the formation of the β chains of haemoglobin and one sickle gene; in the absence of other coincidental disease, the haemoglobin concentration and other red cell indices are normal, the proportion of the total haemoglobin which is Hb-A is greater than that which is Hb-S, and there is a normal proportion of Hb-F.

Sickle-cell disease: the condition resulting from the inheritance of two abnormal allelemorphic genes controlling the formation of the β chains of haemoglobin, at least one of which is the sickle gene; sickle-cell disease includes, therefore, Hb-SS, Hb-SC, Hb-S/β thal and other doubly heterozygous conditions.

Sickle-cell anaemia (Hb-SS): the condition resulting from the inheritance of two sickle genes.

Sickle-cell-haemoglobin C (Hb-SC) disease: the condition resulting from the inheritance of the sickle gene and the Hb-C gene.

Sickle-cell-β-thalassaemia (Hb-S/β thal): the conditions resulting from the inheritance of the sickle gene and one of the various β-thalassaemia genes. For the purposes of this text, these genes are referred to as

(i) β°thal, leading to *complete* suppression of synthesis of β-chains of adult haemoglobin, and

(ii) β^{+}thal, leading to *incomplete* suppression of synthesis of β-chains of adult haemoglobin.

The doubly heterozygous inheritance leads to either Hb-S/β°thal or Hb-S/β^{+}thal.

Sickle-cell-hereditary persistence of fetal haemoglobin (Hb-S/HPFH): the condition resulting from the inheritance of the sickle gene and the gene for HPFH (see below).

Hereditary persistence of fetal haemoglobin (HPFH): a condition characterised by the persistent production of fetal haemoglobin

(Hb-F) into adult life in the absence of any haematological abnormality. There is a uniform distribution of Hb-F in all red cells. There are two main forms, the 'Negro' and the 'Greek'. In Negro heterozygotes, Hb-F is about 25 per cent of the total haemoglobin and the Hb-A_2 is slightly reduced. In the homozygous state, the haemoglobin consists entirely of Hb-F.

Historical introduction. Molecular biology and inheritance

HISTORICAL INTRODUCTION

There is some evidence that sickle-cell disease had been recognised in Africa by black Africans long before the earliest descriptions in the medical literature at the beginning of the twentieth century. Most of this evidence comes from Ghana (Konotey-Ahulu, 1974). It would appear that various ethnic groups in Ghana, including the Twi, Ewe and Ga peoples, identified sickle-cell disease as an entity to the extent of pinpointing some cardinal features, such as the recurrent attacks of pain in the bones and joints, the variable severity of the disease and its familial tendency, but with the parents of affected children appearing normal. Their descriptions were so accurate that in one particular family belonging to the Krobo tribe, Dr Konotey-Ahulu was able to trace the existence of sickle-cell disease in nine generations, dating back to 1670. There is, however, no convincing evidence that these ethnic groups in Ghana related the various symptoms of sickle-cell disease to a disorder of the blood.

Other communities in black Africa, including West Africa, cannot claim this degree of accuracy in the recognition of sickle-cell disease prior to descriptions in modern medical literature. In Nigeria, the largest black African nation, sickle-cell disease apparently remained unrecognised as a distinct disorder by the various ethnic groups until recent times. The Nigerian languages abound with words and phrases which describe various symptoms commonly found in patients with sickle-cell disease. These expressions are however not necessarily specific for this disorder. In the Hausa language for example, expressions such as *rashin jini* (lack of blood), *ciwon ga' bo'bi sai sai* or *amosanin kashi* (recurrent pain in bones and joints) and *rashin kuzari* (lack of energy) are frequently used in relation to sickle-cell disease by patients, their relatives and by traditional healers. However, this current usage of words does not appear to be associated with any long-standing knowledge of sickle-cell disease in the Hausa community. Age-old concepts of *ogbanje* (Ibo) and *abiku* (Yoruba) provide a traditional explanation for recurrent deaths of children in some families. It is just possible that sickle-cell disease may have caused some of these deaths. Interestingly, a disorder in childhood termed *vende wanye* had been recognised for some centuries by the Tivs (one of the largest Nigerian ethnic minorities). Though the descriptions of this disorder may apply to some children suffering from sickle-cell disease, on further investigation *vende wanye* is apparently non-specific and may refer also to other illnesses of childhood, including kwashiokor. Thus, unequivocal and incontrovertible evidence that sickle-cell disease was identified as a distinct abnormality in the traditional societies of Nigeria before its recognition in 'Western' medicine is lacking. However, the earliest descriptions in the Western medical press were inevitably based on features of the disorder as observed in the descendants of Africans (predominantly West Africans) living in the New World.

In 1904, Dr James B. Herrick, a physician practising in Chicago, USA, first noted the presence of red cells which were shaped like a sickle in the blood of an anaemic West Indian medical student. This historic observation linked the 'peculiar and elongated sickle-shaped red blood corpuscles' with severe anaemia (Herrick, 1910). Surprisingly, Herrick preferred to be remembered for his work on coronary thrombosis rather than on the sickling of red cells, a phenomenon he regarded as a 'minor peculiarity'!

As information on the clinical features of sickle-cell disease gradually accumulated over the ensuing years, workers became increasingly preoccupied with the nature and pathogenesis of the disorder. Significant contributions included the work of Emmel (1917), who made pertinent obervations about the familial nature of the disease and suggested that sickling of the red cells might be related to diminished oxygen supply. Huck (1923) noted that sickling was a reversible process. One year later, Sydenstricker (1924) reported additional findings, including the variability in the course of the illness. Hahn and Gillespie (1927) confirmed the intimate relationship between the sickling of red cells and a reduced supply of oxygen, and also demonstrated that sickled red cells could revert to their normal shape when exposed to adequate amounts of oxygen. Significantly, these two workers, as early as 1927, also rightly attributed the defect in the sickling phenomenon to the haemoglobin contained within the red cell and not to the red cell itself. Scriver and Waugh (1930) confirmed *in vivo* Hahn and Gillespie's earlier findings, and demonstrated the formation of sickled cells in situations of stasis in peripheral veins when oxygen tension fell below 5·3 to 6·0 kPa (40 to 45 mmHg).

Early major contributions by Diggs and Ching of Tennessee (1934) included the first detailed post-mortem reports on patients with sickle-cell disease in the United States of America. Five years later, Diggs also reported on certain haematological parameters (haemoglobin content, red cell fragility and detailed morphology of sickled cells) in patients suffering from sickle-cell anaemia (Diggs and Bibb, 1939). They noted for the first time the presence of red cells which were irreversibly sickled even after adequate reoxygenation.

The period between 1940 and 1960 witnessed rapid advances in the understanding of various facets of this disease. Ham and Castle (1940) elaborated on the pathogenesis of the vicious cycle of sickling *in vivo*, that is, sickling results in increased viscosity of blood, which leads to reduced circulation and increased deoxygenation, which in turn causes further sickling. This theoretical concept has been found extremely useful without modification for almost forty years. In the past few years, however, there has been some revaluation. Sherman (1946) observed that deoxygenated sickled cells exhibited optical birefringence, a phenomenon which was not seen in normal red cells. This was probably the first evidence that the deoxygenated form of sickle haemoglobin has an orderly structure.

By the mid 1940s it was clear that there were two classes of individuals whose red cells sickled, (i) the asymptomatic individuals with sickle-cell trait and (ii) the patients with symptoms and sickle-cell anaemia. Neel (1947) suggested that the difference between these two classes of individuals might be explained on the same basis as the difference between major and minor thalassaemia, that is, sickle-cell trait and sickle-cell anaemia were respectively heterozygous and homozygous manifestations of the same gene and not the result of a gene whose effects were of variable severity. Two years later, Beet (1949), a medical officer in the British Colonial Medical Service in Zambia (then Northern Rhodesia), provided convincing evidence of the inherited nature of sickle-cell anaemia and sickle-cell trait. In the same year (1949), Neel provided similar but independent evidence from the United States of America.

The next major milestone in the history of sickle-cell disease was the result of the work of Linus Pauling, twice Nobel Laureate. Antedating Pauling's findings however, was the brilliant speculation by Dr Janet Watson that the sickling phenomenon was related to a different type of adult haemoglobin (Watson et al., 1948). This speculation was based on her observation that infants did not show evidence of sickling until they were about four to six months old. In their classic paper, Pauling *et al.* (1949) reported that, on moving boundary electrophoresis, the haemoglobin of an individual with sickle-cell disease had a different mobility from that of normal adults. Pauling and his colleagues termed the haemoglobin of sickle-cell anaemia patients sickle haemoglobin or haemoglobin S (Hb-S) and the haemoglobin of normal individuals haemoglobin A (Hb-A). They attributed correctly the electrophoretic differences to differences of electrical charge between these two haemoglobins, and Pauling coined the term 'molecular disease' for sickle-cell anaemia. These fundamental studies opened the way to important and exciting discoveries.

Work at Cambridge (England) and New York (United States of America) showed that the solubility of sickle oxyhaemoglobin was normal but that the solubility of 'reduced' sickle haemoglobin was much less than that of 'reduced' normal haemoglobin under physiological conditions of pH, temperature and salt concentration: the deoxygenated red cells of patients with sickle-cell anaemia contained 'reduced' haemoglobin in crystalline form (Perutz and Mitchison, 1950; Perutz *et al.*, 1951). Harris (1950) also described spindle-shaped liquid crystals or tactoids 1 to 15μ long in deoxygenated solutions of sickle haemoglobin.

Using the technique of fingerprinting, Ingram (1956) identified the molecular abnormality of sickle haemoglobin, thereby reinforcing Pauling's original concept of sickle-cell disease as a 'molecular disease'. Thus, in the period of almost half a century between Herrick's original description of sickled red cells and Ingram's identification of the molecular abnormality of Hb-S, the groundwork was laid for the sophisticated and exciting molecular, biological and genetic studies now being carried out in the quest for a answer to the problems of sickle-cell disease.

HAEMOGLOBIN STRUCTURE AND SYNTHESIS

An understanding of the chemical abnormality of Hb-S and the pathogenesis of the sickling phenomenon requires some knowledge of the structure and synthesis of normal haemoglobin. The normal human haemoglobin molecule (mol. wt 64 400) consists of two separate molecules, haem and globin, which are chemically linked.

Globin

Globin is a globular tetrameric protein (mol. wt 61 944) which

accounts for 97·4 per cent of the mass of the haemoglobin molecule. The globin tetramer consists of four polypeptide chains which
are a pair of alpha (α) chains and a pair of non-alpha chains. The
non-alpha chains are the beta (β), gamma (γ) delta (δ), zeta (ζ) or
epsilon (ε) chains. The ζ and ε chains are synthesised during the
first 10 to 12 weeks of fetal life, presumably by erythroid cells de-
rived from the yolk-sac (Fig. 1.1), and are primitive α and β
chains respectively. Synthesis of α and γ chains begins at about
the fourth to fifth week and that of β chains at about the sixth
week of intrauterine life. Production of α chains continues at an
appreciable level throughout pre- and postnatal life. The synthesis
of γ chains is prominent throughout prenatal life but declines
rapidly during the first six months after birth. The synthesis of β
chains is at a relatively low level during intrauterine life but increases significantly in the first few months after birth. The production of small amounts of δ chains begins a few weeks before
birth and increases only slightly after birth. Synthesis of globin
chains is carried out primarily by erythropoietic cells of the liver
and spleen during the first 20 weeks of fetal life, but during the
latter half of pregnancy the fetal bone marrow assumes an increasingly important role as the major erythropoietic organ. After

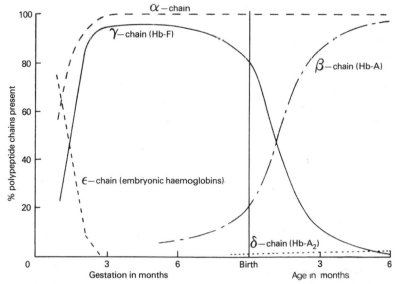

Fig. 1.1 The synthesis of globin chains in intra- and extrauterine life. (From
Huehns, E.R. (1974) The structure and function of haemoglobin: clinical disorders
due to abnormal haemoglobin structure. In *Blood and its Disorders*, eds. Hardisty,
R.M. & Weatherall, D.J. pp. 526–629. Oxford: Blackwell.)

birth, production of globin chains normally occurs entirely in the erythroid cells of the bone marrow.

Like other proteins, the detailed structure of the globin molecule of haemoglobin can be resolved into primary, secondary, tertiary and quarternary structure.

Primary structure. The primary structure refers to the sequence of amino acids in the polypeptide chain. The α chain consists of 141 amino acid residues in sequence (Fig. 1.2). The β chain is slightly longer and consists of 146 amino acid residues (Fig. 1.3); the δ chain also has 146 amino acid residues but differs from the β chain in the nature of 10 of the amino acids. The γ chain has 146 amino acid residues but differs from the β chain in 39 of the residues.

Secondary structure. The stability of the polypeptide chains is achieved by the rotation of segments of each chain into a right-handed (clockwise) spiral or alpha helix (Fig. 1.4) and by hydrogen bonding between amino acids in these helical segments.

Tertiary structure. The β chain is folded on itself to give eight helical segments, named A to H, which are joined by short non-helical segments, named AB, BC, CD, DE etc. (see Fig. 1.4). The helical structure of the α chain is similar to that of the β chain except that it lacks the D-helical segment (see Figs. 1.2 and 1.3). Each constituent amino acid can be designated by its position in a chain or by its position in the appropriately lettered segment; for example, the haem-linked histidine of the β chain may be designated as β 92 or F8.

Quarternary structure. The haemoglobin molecule is assembled when the two α chains and the two non-α chains come together. One α chain makes only a weak contact with the other α chain, but stronger chemical bonds are established between α and β chains (Fig. 1.5). The $\alpha_1 \beta_1$ (and identical $\alpha_2 \beta_2$) contact is firm and stabilises the molecule. The $\alpha_1 \beta_2$ (and identical $\alpha_2 \beta_1$) contact is not rigid and during oxygenation and deoxygenation allows spacial movements which are functionally important.

Haem

The haem moiety (mol. wt 614) forms 2·6 per cent of the mass of the haemoglobin molecule (Fig. 1.6). It is also the prosthetic group of other haemoproteins, including the b-cytochromes, catalase, peroxidase and myoglobin. There are four haem moieties in haemoglobin, each linked to one of the polypeptide chains. Each haem moiety lies in a deep hydrophobic (water-repelling) pocket

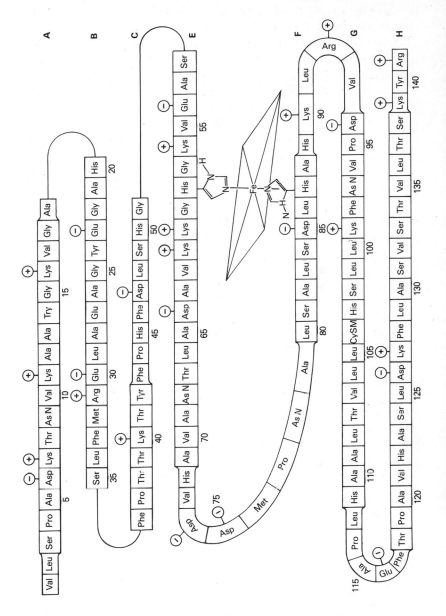

Fig. 1.2 The sequence of 141 amino acid residues in the α chain of haemoglobin. (From Murayama, M. (1971) Molecular mechanism of human red cell (with Hb-S) sickling. In *Molecular aspects of Sickle Cell Hemoglobin*, ed. Nalbandian, R.M. pp. 3–19. Springfield: Thomas.)

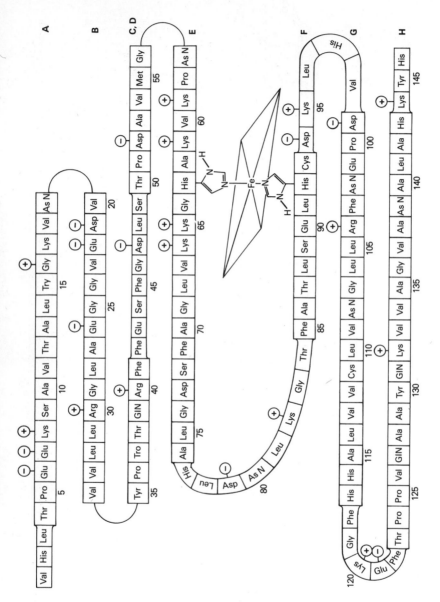

Fig. 1.3 The sequence of 146 amino acid residues in the β chain of haemoglobin. (From Murayama, M. (1971) Molecular mechanism of human red cell (with Hb-S) sickling. In *Molecular Aspects of Sickle Cell Hemoglobin*, ed. Nalbandian, R.M. pp. 3–19. Springfield: Thomas.)

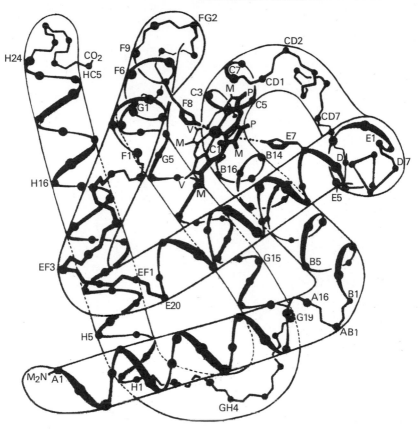

Fig. 1.4 The secondary and tertiary configuration of myoglobin (the monomers of haemoglobin resemble closely myoglobin). (From Dickerson, R.E. (1964) *The Proteins*, 2nd edn., ed. Neurath, H. Vol. 2. New York: Academic Press.)

between the E- and F-helices (see Fig. 1.4). Haem is held firmly in position in the pocket by bonding between the porphyrin ring and the neighbouring amino acids of globin. The iron atom itself is linked chemically to histidine at F8 (the proximal or haem-linked histidine). At the opposite side of the pocket, there is another histidine at E7. This is called the distal histidine, and there is a space between it and the iron atom into which an oxygen molecule fits during oxygenation of haemoglobin.

Haemoglobin function

The tetrameric structure of globin enables the haemoglobin mole-

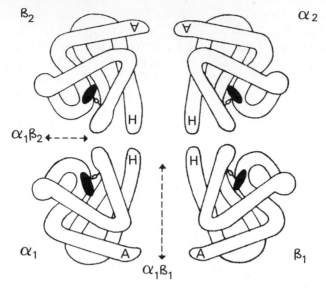

Fig. 1.5 The relationship between α and β chains and haem moieties in the haemoglobin tetramer. (From White, J.M. (1972) The haemoglobinopathies. In *Haematology*, eds. Hoffbrand, A.V. & Lewis, S.M. pp. 184–216. London: Heinemann.)

cule to function as a most effective carrier of oxygen from the lungs to the tissues and of carbon dioxide from the tissues to the lungs.

In the deoxyhaemoglobin state, movement at the $\alpha_1\beta_2$ contact allows the two α β dimers to separate sufficiently for 2,3-diphosphoglycerate (2,3-DPG) to enter between the β chains. The binding of 2,3-DPG stabilises deoxyhaemoglobin, so shifting the

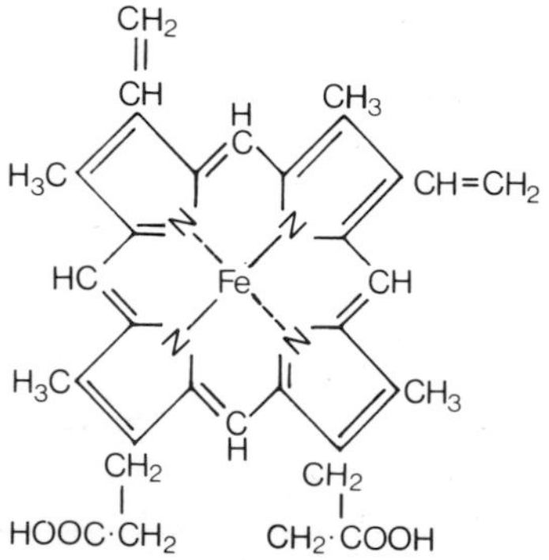

Fig. 1.6 The haem moiety

equilibrium from the oxy- towards the deoxyhaemoglobin form, decreasing oxygen affinity and increasing oxygen release.

When one haem molecule becomes oxygenated, there is a pull on the haem-linked histidine which starts a series of movements and changes in the globin chains, resulting in the two $\alpha\beta$ dimers closing on each other with the exclusion of 2,3-DPG. (The opening of the haemoglobin molecule with deoxygenation and its closing with oxygenation has been called 'paradoxical breathing'.) Oxygen affinity is increased; oxygenation of the next haem moiety and each subsequent haem becomes increasingly easier. This haem–haem in-

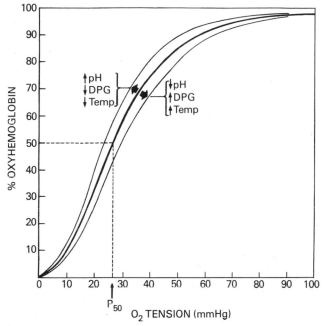

Fig. 1.7 Oxygen dissociation curve of haemoglobin-A and the main factors which influence its position. (From Bunn, H.F., Forget, B.G. & Ranney, H.M. (1977) Oxygen and carbon dioxide transport in the red cell in health and disease. In *Human Hemoglobins*, pp. 60–109. London: Saunders.)

teraction gives the oxygen dissociation curve of haemoglobin its characteristic sigmoid shape (Fig. 1.7). An acid pH, carbon dioxide (acting mainly by reducing pH), increased levels of red cell 2,3-DPG and increased temperatures shift the oxygen dissociation curve to the right (low oxygen affinity and high oxygen release). A high partial pressure of oxygen shifts the curve to the left (high oxygen affinity).

Table 1.1 Globin chain composition of normal haemoglobins in man

Embryonic haemoglobins	
Hb-Gower 1	$\zeta_2\varepsilon_2$
Hb-Gower 2	$\alpha^A_2\varepsilon_2$
Hb-Portland 1	$\zeta_2\eth_2$
Fetal haemoglobin	
Hb-F	$\alpha^A_2\eth^2$
Adult haemoglobins	
Hb-A	$\alpha^A_2\beta^A_2$
Hb-A_2	$\alpha^A_2\delta_2$

Normal human haemoglobins

During the embryonic stages of life, that is, the first 10 to 12 weeks, the haemoglobins found in man are Hb-Gower 1 (probably $\zeta_2\varepsilon_2$) and Hb-Gower 2 ($\alpha_2\varepsilon_2$) (Table 1.1). Production of Hb-F ($\alpha_2\eth_2$) begins early in gestation; at about the sixth week, it constitutes over 30 per cent of the total haemoglobin, and it replaces almost wholly the embryonic haemoglobins by about the twelfth week (see Fig. 1.1).

In the blood of the normal newborn, Hb-F predominates, forming about 90 to 95 per cent of the total haemoglobin; 5 to 10 per cent of Hb-A and trace amounts of Hb-A_2 and Hb-Portland 1 are also found in normal cord blood. After birth, Hb-F levels fall rapidly so that by six months of age, Hb-F contributes less than 1 per cent to the total haemoglobin of a normal infant. After six months of age, over 95 per cent of haemoglobin is Hb-A, less than 4 per cent is Hb-A_2 and less than 1 per cent is Hb-F.

Abnormal haemoglobin synthesis in man

Disorders of synthesis of haemoglobin are invariably inherited and result in either (i) structurally abnormal haemoglobins or (ii) quantitative defects of normal haemoglobins.

The common structurally or qualitatively abnormal haemoglobins show molecular changes in the α or β chains of Hb-A (Table 1.2). Sickle-cell haemoglobin (Hb-S), the commonest abnormal haemoglobin, is formed by the substitution of valine for glutamic acid in the sixth position of the β chain. In Hb-C, the next most common abnormal haemoglobin, lysine is substituted for glutamic acid in the $\beta 6$ position. Other less common but important abnormal haemoglobins affecting blacks in Africa, the Caribbean and the United States of America include the D haemoglobins (D-Ibadan, D-Los Angeles or Punjab, D-Iran) with varying substitutions in the

Table 1.2   Globin chain composition of some abnormal haemoglobins in man

Substitutions on the β chain

Hb-S	$\alpha_2^A \beta_2^S (\alpha_2^A \beta_2^{6\ \text{Glu} \rightarrow \text{Val}})$
Hb-C	$\alpha_2^A \beta_2^C (\alpha_2^A \beta_2^{6\ \text{Glu} \rightarrow \text{Lys}})$
Hb-D-Punjab	$\alpha_2^A \beta_2^D (\alpha_2^A \beta_2^{121\ \text{Glu} \rightarrow \text{Gln}})$
Hb-D-Ibadan	$\alpha_2^A \beta_2^D (\alpha_2^A \beta_2^{87\ \text{Thr} \rightarrow \text{Lys}})$
Hb-O-Arab	$\alpha_2^A \beta_2^O (\alpha_2^A \beta_2^{121\ \text{Glu} \rightarrow \text{Lys}})$
Hb-E	$\alpha_2^A \beta_2^E (\alpha_2^A \beta_2^{26\ \text{Glu} \rightarrow \text{Lys}})$

Substitutions on the α chain

Hb-G-Philadelphia	$\alpha_2^G \beta_2^A (\alpha_2^{68\ \text{Asn} \rightarrow \text{Lys}} \beta_2^A)$

Haemoglobins resulting from impaired synthesis of α chains

Hb-Barts	γ_4
Hb-H	β_4^A

β chain, Hb-O-Arab and Hb-G-Philadelphia, which is an α chain variant. Hb-E, the third most prevalent abnormal haemoglobin in the world, is found mainly in Asia, though it has been described occasionally in blacks. Rare abnormal haemoglobins which occasionally cause clinical disorders include (i) the unstable haemoglobins, (ii) haemoglobins with high or low oxygen affinity and (iii) the M-haemoglobins, which are easily oxidised to abnormal methaemoglobins.

Inherited quantitative defects in the synthesis of globin chains give rise to the thalassaemia syndromes. The α-thalassaemia (α-thal) syndromes arise when there is a genetically-determined impairment of the rate of synthesis of α chains; as a result there is an excess of γ chains in the prenatal period and of β chains in the postnatal period. The excess γ chains form a tetramer called Hb-Barts (γ_4) and excess β chains form Hb-H (β_4) (see Table 1.2). In the β-thalassaemia (β-thal) disorders, the rate of β chain synthesis is impaired with consequent excess formation of α chains, which do not, however, form any haemoglobin tetramer; but there is ineffective erythropoiesis and impaired production of Hb-A.

Haemoglobin-S and the sickling phenomenon

The α chains of Hb-S and Hb-A are structurally identical; the β chains of Hb-S differ from those of Hb-A only in having a hydrophobic valine residue at position 6 instead of glutamic acid. Therefore, the sickling phenomenon and its sequelae must be explained on the basis of this small chemical difference between Hb-S and normal Hb-A. Unfortunately, it has not been possible so far to offer a clear, precise explanation of how this chemical change in the β chains of Hb-S causes sickling under conditions of low oxygen tension. However, significant advances have been made recently in our understanding of the pathogenesis of sickling. Deoxygenated Hb-S and Hb-A have similar physical properties in dilute solutions, but in concentrated solutions deoxy-Hb-S is insoluble and forms a gel, whilst deoxy-Hb-A remains in solution. This difference of solubility forms the physico-chemical basis of sickling.

It is possible to study the sickling process by investigating rates of gel formation in concentrated Hb-S solutions at various oxygen tensions. Deoxy-Hb-S solutions of 24 g/dl (the minimum gelling concentration) or above form gels containing bundles of parallel polymers (fibres) of Hb-S molecules packed in either square or hexagonal lattices. Similar formation and arrangement of polymers are

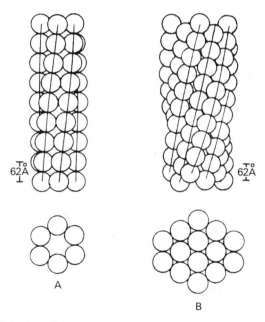

Fig. 1.8 Models of possible structures of polymers of haemoglobin-S. A. Rings of six tetramers stacked to form a hollow microtubule. B. Layers of 14 Hb-S tetramers (4 internal and 10 external) stacked to form a solid fibre. (From Dean, J. & Schechter, A.N. (1978) *New England Journal of Medicine*, **299**, 752–763.)

observed also with deoxygenated sickled red cells. The polymers arrange themselves into paracrystalline (liquid crystal) gels. The polymer may consist of rings of six or eight Hb-S tetramers stacked up to form a microtubular structure with a hollow centre (Fig. 1.8A). Recently, a much more densely packed structure has been described, with 14 Hb-S tetramers comprising an external

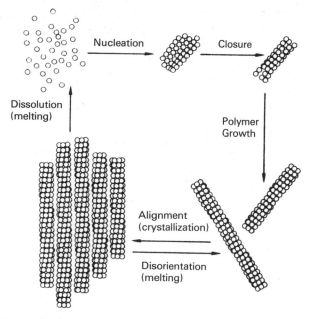

Fig. 1.9 The nucleation, growth and alignment of polymers of deoxyhaemoglobin-S. (From Hofrichter, J. *et al.* (1976) A physical description of hemoglobin S gelation. In *Proceedings of the Symposium on Molecular and Cellular Aspects of Sickle Cell Disease*, Dallas, Texas, December 10, 1975, eds. Hercules, J.I., Cottam, G.L., Waterman, M.R. & Schechter, A.N. pp. 185–223. Bethesda, Maryland: US Department of Health, Education and Welfare.)

arrangement of 10 tetramers and an internal group of 4 tetramers in each layer of the polymer (Fig. 1.8B). It is possible that other models may yet be described.

Recent studies into the kinetics of formation of Hb-S polymers or gels using physicochemical methods suggest three phases: (i) nucleation, (ii) growth and (iii) alignment (Fig. 1.9). In the nucleation phase, Hb-S tetramers are believed to associate with each other to form aggregates of increasing size; when this nucleus reaches a critical size, the growth phase occurs, during which free haemoglobin tetramers are rapidly added on to form long polymers. Subsequent alignment of the polymers in an orderly manner then follows.

Participation of other normal and abnormal haemoglobins with Hb-S in gel formation is variable. Normal Hb-A interacts with Hb-S to only a slight extent, while Hb-F does not participate in gel formation when mixed with Hb-S; this may explain in part the inhibitory effect of Hb-F on the sickling process *in vivo*. Some abnormal haemoglobins, such as Hb-C and Hb-O-Arab, show considerable interaction with Hb-S in gel formation; thus, these two abnormal haemoglobins participate to a marked extent during sickling *in vivo* when present with Hb-S in red cells.

Intracellular polymerisation within the sickled cell leads to functional abnormalities in the red cell membrane which result in increased potassium (K^+) leak out of and increased sodium movement into the red cell. There is also an increase in intracellular calcium ions (Ca^{2+}). Repeated sickling and unsickling leads to a net loss of water and K^+ from the cell; this results in a dehydrated red cell with increase in intracellular haemoglobin concentration, which further enhances the intracellular formation of gels of Hb-S. Reoxygenation of sickled cells *in vivo* or *in vitro* reverses the sickling process, but a variable proportion of cells remains sickled even after adequate reoxygenation and subsequent depolymerisation of Hb-S. Such cells are termed irreversibly sickled cells (ISC). The excessive intracellular accumulation of Ca^{2+} is probably responsible for the defects associated with ISC formation.

Genetic control of haemoglobin synthesis

The synthesis of structurally normal haemoglobin chains is determined by allelic genes situated on autosomal chromosomes. It is generally accepted that there are single β and δ chain genetic loci inherited from both parents but that the α chain locus is duplicated so that an individual has four genes controlling α chain synthesis. The ઠ chain structural genes are multiple, possibly two or three. The β, δ and ઠ chain genes are probably all linked on the same chromosome, but the α chain gene is on a different chromosome.

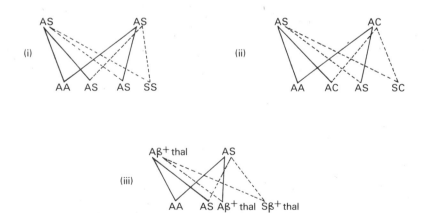

Fig. 1.10 The inheritance of sickle-cell disease. (i) Sickle-cell anaemia (Hb-SS). (ii) Sickle-cell-haemoglobin C disease. (iii) Sickle-cell β⁺ thalassaemia (inheritance of Sickle-cell β° thalassaemia is similar).

Inheritance of haemoglobin-S

Inheritance of Hb-S results from an abnormal β^s gene (or sickle gene) which codes for valine instead of glutamic acid at position 6 in the β chain. The α chain gene is normal. The sickle gene is possibly the result of a single point mutation in the DNA codon for glutamic acid. This would give rise theoretically to an abnormal messenger RNA (mRNA) base triplet of guanosine-uridine-guanosine (GUG) which codes for valine, rather than the normal mRNA base triplet of guanosine-adenosine-guanosine (GAG) which codes for glutamic acid in the β 6 position. The inheritance of the sickling disorders follows simple Mendelian laws.

Sickle-cell trait. When an individual inherits a sickle gene from one parent and a normal haemoglobin (Hb-A) gene from the other parent, both gene products are expressed and the red cells contain both Hb-A and Hb-S, but the amount of Hb-A is greater than Hb-S. Such an individual is said to have sickle-cell trait (Hb-AS) (Fig. 1.10).

Sickle-cell anaemia. An individual who inherits sickle genes from both parents is a sickle cell homozygote who suffers from sickle-cell anaemia (Hb-SS) (Fig. 1.10). The only major adult haemoglobin formed is Hb-S, but the red cells contain in addition variable amounts of Hb-F and normal proportions of Hb-A_2.

Interaction between haemoglobin-S and other β chain abnormalities

If an individual inherits a sickle gene from one parent and another abnormal β chain gene which results in the formation of a second abnormal haemoglobin, that individual is said to be a double hetero-zygote. No normal β chains and hence no normal adult haemoglo-bin can be produced. If the second abnormal haemoglobin partici-pates in gel formation when mixed with Hb-S, there is said to be interaction, and the subject suffers from a form of sickle-cell dis-ease. The commonest haemoglobin interacting with Hb-S is Hb-C.

Sickle-cell-haemoglobin C disease. The inheritance of a sickle gene from one parent and a Hb-C gene (β^c gene) from the other parent gives rise to the doubly heterozygous individual whose red cells contain both Hb-S and Hb-C (see Fig. 1.10). Hb-C participates with Hb-S in gel formation so that the subject has a sickle-cell disease, Hb-SC disease, which is generally milder than Hb-SS.

Sickle-cell-β-thalassaemias. Sickle-cell disease states result also from the inheritance of the sickle gene from one parent and a β-thal gene from the other parent (see Fig. 1.10).

The β^+-thal gene partially suppresses the synthesis of β chains. A double heterozygote (Hb-S/β^+-thal) individual synthesises reduced amounts of Hb-A, and the red cells contain both Hb-S and Hb-A, but the amount of Hb-S is greater than that of Hb-A. Gelling of Hb-S occurs at low oxygen tensions, but to a less extent than in Hb-SS. The patient suffers from a mild form of sickle-cell disease.

The $\beta°$-thal gene suppresses completely β chain synthesis. The doubly heterozygous individual (Hb-S/$\beta°$-thal) is unable to synthesise any Hb-A, and the red cells contain only Hb-S, with some Hb-F and Hb-A_2. Hb-S/$\beta°$-thal double heterozygotes resemble Hb-SS homozygotes both in their haemoglobin composition and clinically, but there are some differences which will be described in later chapters.

Inheritance of haemoglobin-S and α *chain abnormalities*
The genetic control of the α chains of globin is not linked to that of the β chains. An α chain variant (or even two) may be inherited by subjects who are also heterozygous (Hb-AS) or homozygous (Hb-SS) for Hb-S. Haemoglobins with abnormalities of the α chains do not interact with Hb-S in gel formation, but rather their coincidental inheritance may sometimes ameliorate the clinical course of sickle-cell disease.

Haemoglobin-G-Philadelphia. Inheritance of the α chain variant Hb-G-Philadelphia with sickle-cell trait allows the production of four major haemoglobins, Hb-A ($\alpha_2^A \beta_2^A$), Hb-G-Philadelphia ($\alpha_2^G \beta_2^A$), Hb-S ($\alpha_2^A \beta_2^S$) and the hybrid Hb-S/G ($\alpha_2^G \beta_2^S$). The clinical condition is that of Hb-AS. Inheritance with sickle-cell anaemia allows the production of three major haemoglobins (Hb-S, Hb-G-Philadelphia and Hb-S/G); the clinical condition of Hb-SS is unaltered. Haematological diagnosis is discussed in Chapter 3.

α-*Thalassaemia.* There are two α-thal genes affecting the duplicated α chain gene loci.

(i) With the α-thal 1 gene, synthesis of α chains is suppressed on both loci: in heterozygous inheritance ($--/\alpha\alpha$) two loci are active and two are inactive, in homozygous inheritance ($--/--$) all loci are inactive.

(ii) With the α-thal 2 gene, synthesis of α chains is suppressed at one locus only: in heterozygous inheritance ($-\alpha/\alpha\alpha$) three loci are active and in homozygous inheritance ($-\alpha/-\alpha$) only two loci are active.

The α-thal 2 gene is relatively common amongst West Africans and those of West African descent. The α-thal 1 gene is rare in Africa but is seen commonly in the Far East.

The inheritance of α-thal 2 and sickle-cell trait by the same subject results in a relatively slow rate of production of Hb-S and a low proportion (even less than 25 per cent) of Hb-S in the red cells. The inheritance of homozygous α-thal 2 with Hb-SS has an ameliorating effect on the clinical course of sickle-cell anaemia. Heterozygous inheritance of α-thal 2 with Hb-SS does not appear to influence the severity of sickle-cell anaemia.

Population genetics
If the incidence of sickle-cell trait is known amongst the adults of the population, it is simple to calculate the proportion of infants which will be born into that population with each genotype, Hb-AA, Hb-AS and Hb-SS. For example, if 20 per cent of the adults have Hb-AS and 80 per cent have Hb-AA, then 10 per cent of the total genes are sickle-genes; this may be expressed as a proportion of 1·0, that is, the frequency of the gene for Hb-A is 0·90 and that of the sickle gene 0·10. The expected distribution of genotypes in the newborn follows the Hardy-Weinberg law, $a^2 + 2as + s^2 = 1·0$, where a is the frequency of the gene for Hb-A and s is the frequency of the sickle-gene.

$a^2 = 0·90^2 = 0·81$; 81 per cent of newborn will be Hb-AA.
$2as = 2 \times 0·90 \times 0·10 = 0·18$; 18 per cent of newborn will be Hb-AS.
$s^2 = 0·10^2 = 0·01$; 1 per cent of newborn will be Hb-SS.

The same principle can be applied if more than one abnormal haemoglobin is found in the population; for example, if the adult population are Hb-AA 72 per cent, Hb-AS 24 per cent and Hb-AC 4 per cent, gene frequencies are a = 0·86, s = 0·12 and c = 0·02. The genotype distribution in the next generation will be according to the equation:

$a^2 + 2as + 2ac + 2sc + s^2 + c^2 = 1·0$.
$a^2 = 0·86^2 = 0·74$; 74 per cent of newborn will be Hb-AA.
$2as = 2 \times 0·86 \times 0·12 = 0·21$; 21 per cent of newborn will be Hb-AS.
$2ac = 2 \times 0·86 \times 0.02 = 0·03$; 3 per cent of newborn will be Hb-AC.
$2sc = 2 \times 0·12 \times 0·02 = 0·0048$; 0·48 per cent of newborn will be Hb-SC.
$s^2 = 0·12^2 = 0·0144$; 1·44 per cent of newborn will be Hb-SS.
$c^2 = 0·02^2 = 0.0004$; 0·04 per cent of newborn will be Hb-CC.

The knowledge that between 1 and 2 per cent of all infants born in the community have sickle-cell disease is invaluable in planning health strategy. As the general standard of living and of medical care improves, these children will live in increasing numbers and to greater ages. They will present a large burden on the available resources, but it is reasonable to hope that, in the not too distant future, current intensive research will bear fruit and provide permanent solutions to the problems of sickle-cell disease.

REFERENCES

Beet, E.A. (1949) The genetics of the sickle-cell trait in a Bantu tribe. *Annals of Eugenics*, 14, 279–284.

Diggs, L.W. & Bibb, J. (1939) The erythrocyte in sickle-cell anemia: morphology, size, hemoglobin content, fragility and sedimentation rate. *Journal of the American Medical Association*, 112, 695–700.

Diggs, L.W. & Ching, R.E. (1934) Pathology of sickle cell anemia. *Southern Medical Journal*, 27, 839–845.

Emmel, V.E. (1917) A study of the erythrocytes in a case of severe anemia with elongated and sickle-shaped red blood corpuscles. *Archives of Internal Medicine*, 20, 586–598.

Hahn, E.V. & Gillespie, E.B. (1927) Sickle cell anemia. *Archives of Internal Medicine*, 39, 233–254.

Ham, T.H. & Castle, W.B. (1940) Relation of increased hypotonic fragility and of erythrostasis to the mechanism of hemolysis in certain anemias. *Transactions of the Association of American Physicians*, 55, 127–132.

Harris, J.W. (1950) Studies on the destruction of red blood cells. VIII. Molecular orientation in sickle cell hemoglobin solutions. *Proceedings of the Society for Experimental Biology and Medicine*, 75, 197–201.

Herrick, J.B. (1910) Peculiar elongated and sickle-shaped red blood corpuscles in a case of severe anemia. *Archives of Internal Medicine*, 6, 517–521.

Huck, J.G. (1923) Sickle cell anemia. *Bulletin of Johns Hopkins Hospital*, 34, 335–344.

Ingram, V.M. (1956) A specific chemical difference between the globins of normal human and sickle-cell anaemia haemoglobin. *Nature*, 178, 792–794.

Konotey-Ahulu, F.I.D. (1974) The sickle cell diseases: clinical manifestations including the 'sickle crisis'. *Archives of Internal Medicine*, 133, 611–619.

Neel, J.V. (1947) The clinical detection of the genetic carriers of inherited disease. *Medicine*, 26, 115–153.

Neel, J.V. (1949) The inheritance of sickle cell anemia. *Science*, 110, 64–66.

Pauling, L., Itano, H.A., Singer, S.J. & Wells, I.C. (1949) Sickle cell anemia, a molecular disease. *Science*, 110, 543–548.

Perutz, M.F. & Mitchison, J.M. (1950) State of haemoglobin in sickle-cell anaemia. *Nature*, 166, 677–679.

Perutz, M.F., Liquori, A.M. & Eirich, F. (1951) X-ray and solubility studies of the haemoglobin of sickle-cell anaemia patients. *Nature*, 167, 929–931.

Scriver, J.B. & Waugh, T.R. (1930) Studies on a case of sickle-cell anaemia. *Canadian Medical Association Journal*, 23, 375–380.

Sherman, I.J. (1946) The sickling phenomenon, with special reference to the differentiation of sickle-cell anemia from the sickle-cell trait. *Bulletin of Johns Hopkins Hospital*, 67, 309–324.

Sydenstricker, V.P. (1924) Further observations on sickle cell anemia. *Journal of the American Medical Association*, 83, 12–17.

Watson, J., Stahman, A.W. & Bilello, F.P. (1948) Significance of the paucity of sickle cells in newborn Negro infants. *American Journal of the Medical Sciences*, 215, 419–423.

FURTHER READING

Bunn, H.F., Forget, B.G. & Ranney, H.M. (1977) *Human Hemoglobins*. Philadelphia: Saunders.

Dean, J. & Schechter, A.N. (1978) Sickle-cell anemia: molecular and cellular bases of therapeutic approaches. *New England Journal of Medicine*, **299**, 752–763.

Hercules, J.I., Cottam, G.L., Waterman, M.R. & Schechter, A.N. (eds.) (1976) *Proceedings of the Symposium on Molecular and Cellular Aspects of Sickle Cell Disease*. Washington, DC: US Department of Health, Education and Welfare.

Sickle-cell trait. Genetic counselling

SICKLE-CELL TRAIT

The individual who inherits one sickle-gene from one parent only is said to have sickle-cell trait (Hb-AS). After the first six months of life, the red cells contain both Hb-A and Hb-S; the Hb-S contributes usually 25 per cent to 45 per cent of the total haemoglobin concentration, but lower proportions of Hb-S are observed in subjects who inherit α-thal as well as sickle-cell trait. If the proportion of Hb-S is greater than 45 per cent, or if there is more Hb-S than Hb-A, the correct diagnosis is probably Hb-S/β^+ thal and *not* Hb-AS.

In absence of coincidental disease, the subject with sickle-cell trait is not anaemic and is haematologically normal except for the presence of Hb-S. Sickle-cell trait is not associated with any shortening of life span.

Sickle-cell trait and malaria

Sickle-cell trait is seen at an incidence of between 20 and 40 per cent in the black populations of Africa (Fig. 2.1). It occurs also at high incidence in certain areas of the Middle East (Arabia and Iran), the Mediterranean basin (Turkey, Greece, Italy and Sicily) and the Indian subcontinent. From these sites, it has been spread by the slave-trade, and by emigration to the Caribbean and the American mainland, where it occurs in about 10 per cent of the black population (Lehmann and Huntsman, 1972), to Europe (especially Britain) and to Australia.

To explain this high frequency, it has been argued that there must be either a high rate of mutation replacing in each generation the sickle genes lost through the nearly complete failure of homozygotes (Hb-SS) to reproduce, or a biological advantage for the heterozygotes (Hb-AS). There is no evidence that the sickle gene is being maintained by a high rate of mutation; in fact, it is possible that this mutation has occurred once only in the history of human

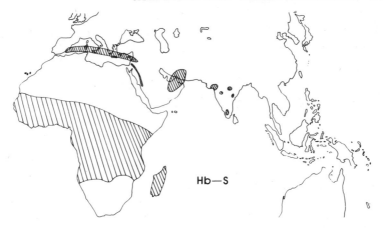

Fig. 2.1 The areas of the world where haemogloin-S occurs commonly: migration and the slave trade have carried the gene to the Americas, northern Europe including Britain, Australia and elsewhere.

evolution. On the other hand, there is a considerable body of evidence that the sickle gene has spread and reached high frequencies in certain populations because the heterozygotes (Hb-AS) enjoy a partial protection against the effects of severe *Plasmodium falciparum* malaria.

Differential survival
The prevalence of sickle-cell trait in African populations rises from the time of birth until about five years of age; for example, in Garki, Kano State in northern Nigeria, the prevalence rose from 23 per cent in the newborn to 29 per cent at five years of age, after which there was no further change (Fleming *et al.*, 1979). The differential of survival Hb-AS/Hb-AA was 1.29, or in other words, the sickle-cell trait individuals had a 29 per cent advantage over those with normal haemoglobin.

The survival advantage of sickle-cell trait, and hence its prevalence, rises with the increasing intensity of transmission of malaria in Africa. However, when transmission is very high and continuous (holoendemic malaria), immunity is actively acquired earlier than where transmission is intermittent in intensity (hyperendemic malaria). As a result, the period of advantage enjoyed by children with Hb-AS may be longer and the frequency of the sickle gene may be higher in some hyperendemic than in holoendemic areas. Sickle-cell trait has an incidence of about 30 per cent in northern parts of Nigeria, where malaria is hyperendemic, and only 24 per cent where malaria is holoendemic in the southern forests.

Malarial parasitology
The newborn infant is protected partially against malaria by the action of IgG antibodies derived from the mother and by the presence of Hb-F. *P. falciparum* parasitaemia becomes frequent and intense from the age of six months; after that age, there are significantly lower frequencies and, more importantly, lower densities of *P. falciparum* in children with sickle-cell trait than in children with normal haemoglobin. This period of parasitological advantage continues until immunity is actively acquired around five years of age; in older children and adults, parasite frequencies and densities are the same in Hb-AS and Hb-AA. The consequences of partial protection against intense *P. falciparum* parasitaemia is shown most clearly by the almost complete absence of Hb-AS children amongst those dying from cerebral malaria.

It should be realised, however, that protection is partial and that children with Hb-AS may have even severe infections with *P. falciparum*. No significant protect against *P. malariae* or *P. ovale* has been observed.

Differential fertility
Resistance against malaria is diminished during normal pregnancy, especially first pregnancies. There is an increase of frequency and density of *P. falciparum* parasitaemia, and this leads to maternal anaemia and parasitic infection of the placenta from the second trimester onwards; these lead in turn to a high frequency of abortion, premature delivery, low birthweight and perinatal mortality. Women with sickle-cell trait have less intense *P. falciparum* parasitaemia and less anaemia in pregnancy than women with normal haemoglobin. However, this parasitological advantage is slight and is not sufficient to result in better reproductive efficiency in women with sickle-cell trait.

Mechanisms for limiting parasitaemia
Recently developed systems of continuous culture of *P. falciparum* in human red cells have thrown light on the mechanisms by which malarial parasitaemia is limited in subjects with sickle-cell trait. Two possible mechanisms are suggested, (i) the sickling of parasitised red cells and their removal by the reticuloendothelial system, and (ii) the inhibition of growth of the malaria parasite in red cells containing Hb-S.

In the early parts of the cycle of *P. falciparum*, small parasites circulate in the red cells of the peripheral blood. These conditions were simulated for cultures of *P. falciparum* in Hb-AA and Hb-AS blood: when the proportion of oxygen was reduced to 30–50 per cent, there was enhanced sickling of those Hb-AS red cells which contained parasites, due presumably to the consumption of oxygen by the parasites themselves. It was postulated that the parasitised and sickled red cells would then be removed *in vivo* by the reticuloendothelial system, so limiting the extent of the infection (Luzzatto *et al.*, 1970; Roth *et al.*, 1978).

The last 12 hours of the erythrocyte cycle of *P. falciparum* are spent in deep tissues at low oxygen tension. It has been demonstrated in cultures at low oxygen tension (5 per cent oxygen at 4·65 k Pa/35 mmHg) that there is reduced invasion of red cells and an inhibition of growth of mature parasite forms in red cells containing Hb-S. The physicochemical changes in the deoxygenated Hb-S molecule were sufficient to account for the inhibition, and the actual process of sickling did not contribute (Friedman, 1978; Pasvol *et al.*, 1978).

Thus, preferential sickling of parasitised red cells in the early part of the cycle of *P. falciparum* and inhibition of growth by the gelling of Hb-S in the late part of the cycle may both contribute to limiting parasitaemia.

The other common abnormalities of haemoglobin synthesis (Hbs-C,D and E, β-thal and α-thal) are also found in parts of the world where malaria is, or was, endemic (Figs. 2.2, 2.3, 2.4). This geographical coincidence is evidence that these genes too confer some protection against malaria, but the mechanisms are still wholly obscure.

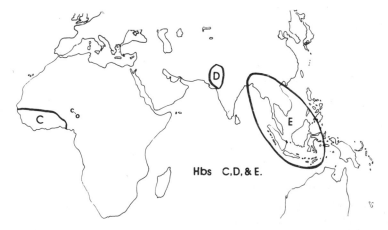

Fig. 2.2 The areas of the world where haemoglobin-C, D-Punjab (also called D-Los Angeles) and E occur commonly.

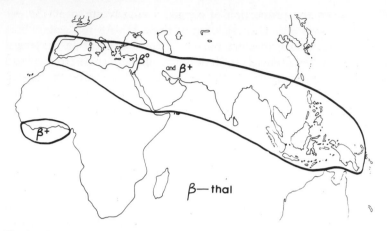

Fig. 2.3 The areas of the world where the β-thalassaemias occur commonly.

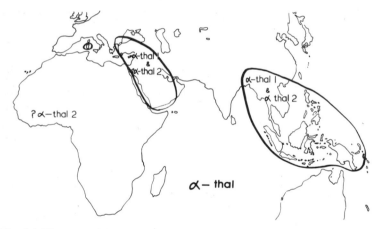

Fig. 2.4 The areas of the world where the α-thalassaemias occur commonly. The frequency and distribution of α-thal 2 in Africa is still largely uncertain.

Humoral immunity in sickle-cell trait

Concentrations of immunoglobulins and titres of antibodies are the same in Hb-AA and Hb-AS persons in non-malarial countries. However, when *P. falciparum* is endemic, there are on average lower concentrations of immunoglobulins (especially IgM) and lower titres of antibodies specific against *P. falciparum* in Hb-AS than in Hb-AA subjects. There differences are most probably the result of sickle-cell trait persons receiving less malarial antigenic stimulus (Cornille-Brøgger *et al.*, 1979). The difference in levels of antibodies persists and increases throughout life, although parasitological differences cannot be demonstrated after about five years of age.

Splenomegaly and sickle-cell trait. In agreement with there being a smaller load of malarial antigen and less stimulus to the production of antibodies, the size of the spleen is on average smaller in Hb-AS children than in those with normal haemoglobin. In later life, sickle-cell trait affords almost complete protection against the development of the tropical splenomegaly syndrome (TSS), a condition which occurs in patients with acquired immunity to malaria and is characterised by gross enlargement of the liver and spleen, lymphoid hyperplasia, and overproduction of IgM and antibodies specific against *P. falciparum* (Bryceson *et al.*, 1976).

Antimeningococcal antibodies. Immune responses are suppressed by acute malaria so that it might be predicted that children with sickle-cell trait would mount better than normal immune responses to other infections. This has been demonstrated in the case of a better antibody response to meningococcal vaccine (Greenwood, B.M., personal communication).

Possible disadvantages of sickle-cell trait

Many symptoms, conditions and complications have been claimed to arise from the inheritance of sickle-cell trait, but there is not more than the merest anecdotal evidence to support such reports (Sears, 1978). The essential normality of sickle-cell trait should be emphasised always to the carriers of the trait and their relatives. The only exception is an impairment of renal function, resulting probably from sickling of red cells in the hypertonic, acidotic and hypoxic conditions of the renal medulla. Individuals with normal haemoglobin conserve water and produce a more concentrated urine during hot and dry weather, but this ability is lost to some extent by subjects with sickle-cell trait (Taylor *et al..* 1978). The sickling of red cells and infarction in the kidneys of Hb-AS subjects can lead to papillary necrosis and increased frequencies of haematuria, bacteriuria and pyelonephritis, especially during pregnancy. In one American series, 13·9 per cent of Hb-AS women had significant bacteriuria during pregnancy, a frequency twice that of the control group (Whalley *et al.* 1964).

It has also been reported that in Nigerian women with Hb-AS, there was an increased risk of death of the fetus in the presence of severe anoxic complications of pregnancy (Platt, 1971).

Sickle-cell trait and aviation
Before haemoglobin electrophoresis became an established techni-

que, the diagnosis of sickle-cell trait was made usually when the individual was healthy but there was sickling of the red cells in suspension with a reducing agent, such as sodium metabisulphite (the sickling test — see Ch. 3). There were several reports of positive sickling tests in individuals who had suffered splenic infarcts triggered by hypoxia during travel in unpressurised aircraft. Many of these persons had undoubtedly various forms of sickle-cell disease, including Hb-SC and Hb-S/β^+ thal. There is no reported instance of splenic infarction induced by flying in any normal individual with sickle-cell trait proven by haemoglobin electrophoresis. In the past twenty-five years, the medical literature has not contained any authenticated report of complications associated with air travel and sickle-cell trait.

It is agreed generally that persons with sickle-cell trait should be permitted to travel freely as passengers on commercial and other aircraft. Some authorities are unwilling to enrol sickle-cell trait subjects as pilots or pilots-in-training. It is our opinion that this restriction is mistaken and is not supported by any physiological or medical observations. It is important, however, to ensure that the diagnosis of sickle-cell trait is correct and that the potential pilot does not have a mild form of sickle-cell anaemia, for example Hb-S/β^+ thal. Following the recommendations of the International Civil Aviation Organization (ICAO) (1974), an individual may be enrolled as a pilot if he is in good health and has sickle-cell trait. Sickle-cell trait should be strictly defined by the following criteria:

1. electrophoresis shows two bands in the positions of the Hb-A and Hb-S
2. the Hb-S solubility test confirms the presence of Hb-S
3. Hb-S does not exceed 45 per cent of the total haemoglobin
4. Hb-F is less than 1 per cent and Hb-A$_2$ less than 4 per cent of the total haemoglobin
5. other haematological measurements give normal results.

GENETIC COUNSELLING

There are three situation to be considered: (i) population counselling, (ii) genetic counselling to individuals before marriage and (iii) counselling to couples after marriage.

Population counselling. Mass screening of a population in which the sickle-cell gene is common is possible and desirable only in a country which can afford the cost and in which there is a widespread understanding of sickle-cell disease and its inheritance. It allows young people to learn that they have sickle-cell trait, and this knowledge may influence their choice of marital partner. On the other hand, two people with sickle-cell trait may decide to marry and have children knowing that each child has a one-in-four chance of having sickle-cell anaemia (see Fig. 1.10). Where antenatal diagnosis of sickle-cell disease and the choice of termination of pregnancy are available (see Ch. 9), it may be anticipated that more sickle-cell trait couples will decide to proceed with marriage.

The disadvantages of mass screening have been demonstrated in the United States of America. Unless it is made clear to the individual that sickle-cell trait is entirely harmless, unnecessary anxiety can be caused. Furthermore, some sickle-cell trait carriers have been quite unjustifiably placed at disadvantage by employers and by life insurance companies. Any mass screening programme must include education of the whole population as to the benign nature of sickle-cell trait.

Genetic counselling before marriage. In Africa, an understanding of sickle-cell disease is confined at present to a small proportion of even the well educated. Screening for sickle-cell trait should be available to those who request it. If two people wishing to marry are both sickle-cell trait, or if one has Hb-AS and the other another β chain abnormality, such as Hb-AC, the counsellor's role is confined to giving information as to the nature of sickle-cell disease and its inheritance. The decisions a couple make once they have that information are entirely their own responsibility.

Genetic counselling after marriage. Advice is sought in Africa far more often after marriage, when there are already one or more affected children in the family. Again, the counsellor's role is to inform, and to advise on birth control if the couple decide they do not wish to have more children. A three-and-a-half year follow up of 45 Nigerian families in Ibadan showed that following counselling, one third practised birth control and one fifth had divorced or the husband had taken another (polygamous) wife, but almost half of the couples had taken no action (Adeyokunnu and Adeyeri, the husband had taken another (polygamous) wife, but almost half of the couples had taken no action (Adeyokunnu and Adeyeri, 1978).

It should be remembered that there can be marriages between patients with sickle-cell disease (Hb-SC, Hb-SS, Hb-S/β^+thal or Hb-S/β °thal) and individuals with sickle-cell trait, Hb-AC or some other β chain abnormality. These matings are becoming increasingly frequent due to the increased survival and wellbeing of patients with sickle-cell disease, who are receiving better medical care in many parts of the world: there can be marriage even between two patients with sickle-cell disease. The possible genotypes of children resulting from these matings are worked out easily from Mendelian principles, and the couples advised accordingly.

THE FUTURE OF THE SICKLE GENE

There are at least four factors which are likely to affect the frequency of the sickle gene in Africa in the future: (i) the control of *P. falciparum* malaria, (ii) improved survival and health of those with sickle-cell disease, (iii) genetic counselling and (iv) intermarriage with other populations.

In the event of the transmission of malaria being interrupted throughout the continent of Africa, sickle-cell trait would no longer confer advantage. If it is assumed that Hb-SS subjects remain with extremely low or no reproductive ability, then the frequency of the sickle gene will decline with every subsequent generation. Under

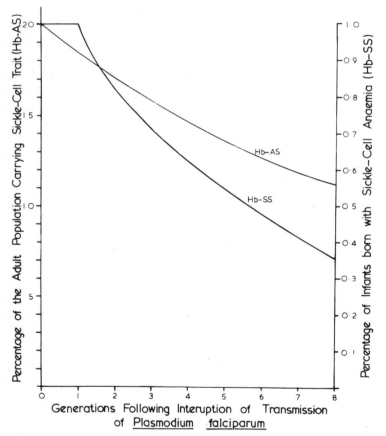

Fig. 2.5 The anticipated decline of the prevalence of sickle-cell trait (Hb-AS) in the adult population, and of sickle-cell anaemia (Hb-SS) in the newborn, in a population freed from *P. falciparum* malaria. Initially, 20 per cent of adults carried sickle-cell trait, and 1 per cent of newborn had sickle-cell anaemia. After eight generations free from malaria, the figures will be 11·2 per cent and 0·35 per cent respectively.

these conditions, the descendants of an initial population with 20 per cent sickle-cell trait will show only about 11 per cent in eight generations (Fig. 2.5). The incidence of Hb-SS in the newborn will fall from 1 per cent to 0·35 per cent in eight generations, or in about 200 years. The decline of the frequency of the sickle gene amongst Black Americans has been of this order since they left the African continent.

Improvements in the standard of living and medical care will lead to more patients with sickle-cell disease living to adulthood and having children. This will lead to a slower rate of decline in a population which is free from malaria. Effective genetic counselling will have complex results on the population. Immediately, it should reduce the number of infants born with sickle-cell disease, but it will also increase the proportion born with sickle-cell trait. Because there will be more with Hb-AS, there will be a tendency for more sickle-cell disease in subsequent generations. Hence, genetic counselling may benefit individual families but will slow the rate of decline of the frequency of the sickle gene in the whole population once freed from malaria.

REFERENCES

Adeyokunnu, A.A. & Adeyeri, C.L.K. (1978) Genetic counselling in sickle cell disease, Ibadan (Nigeria) experience. *Tropical Pediatrics and Environmental Child Health*, **24**, 148–151.
Bryceson, A.D.M., Fleming, A.F. & Edington, G.M. (1976) Splenomegaly in northern Nigeria. *Acta Tropica*, **33**, 185–214.
Cornille-Brøgger, R., Fleming, A.F., Kagan, I., Matsushima, T. & Molineaux, L. (1979) Abnormal haemoglobins in the Sudan Savanna of Nigeria. II. Immunological response to malaria in normals and subjects with sickle-cell trait. *Annals of Tropical Medicine and Parasitology*, **73**, 173–184.
Fleming, A.F., Storey, J., Molineaux, L., Iroko, E.A. & Attai, E.D.E. (1979) Abnormal haemoglobins in the Sudan Savanna of Nigeria. I. Prevalence of haemoglobins and relationships between sickle-cell trait, malaria and survival. *Annals of Tropical Medicine and Parasitology*, **73**, 161–172.
Friedman, M.J. (1978) Erythrocyte mechanisms of sickle-cell resistance to malaria. *Proceedings of the National Academy of Science of the United States of America*, **75**, 1994–1997.
International Civil Aviation Organization (1974) *Manual of Civil Aviation Medicine*, ICAO Document 8984–AN/895.
Lehmann, H. & Huntsman, R.G. (1972) *Man's Haemoglobins*, 2nd edn. Amsterdam: North-Holland.
Luzzatto, L., Nwachuku-Jarrett, E.S. & Reddy, S. (1970) Increased sickling of parasitized erythrocytes as mechanism of resistance against malaria in the sickle-cell trait. *Lancet*, **i**, 319–322.
Pasvol, G., Weatherall, D.J. & Wilson, R.J.M. (1978) Cellular mechanism for the protective effect of haemoglobin S against *P. falciparum* malaria. *Nature*, **274**, 701–703.
Platt, H.S. (1971) Effect of maternal sickle-cell trait on perinatal mortality. *British Medical Journal*, **iv**, 334–336.

Roth, E.F., Friedman, M., Ueda, Y., Tellez, I., Trager, W. & Nagel, R.L. (1978) Sickling rates of human AS red cells infected with *Plasmodium falciparum* malaria. *Science*, **202**, 650–652.

Sears, D.A. (1978) The morbidity of sickle cell trait. *American Journal of Medicine*, **64**, 1021–1036.

Taylor, G.O., Oyediran, A.B.O.O. & Saliu, I. (1978) Effects of haemoglobin electrophoretic pattern and seasonal changes on urine concentration in young adult Nigerian males. *African Journal of Medical Sciences*, **7**, 201–205.

Whalley, P.J., Martin, F.G. & Pritchard, J.A. (1964) Sickle cell trait and urinary tract infection during pregnancy. *Journal of the American Medical Association*, **189**, 903–906.

The essential laboratory investigation of sickle-cell disease

Since the early days of the study of sickle-cell disease, the clinical laboratory has played an important role in its accurate diagnosis and management. This has resulted in over 300 abnormal haemoglobins being recognized and also in a profusion in the number, type and variation of tests that are now used. Each laboratory usually has its own choice set for which it claims superiority, and several commercial kits are now available. In this section, we review the essential methods for the diagnosis or confirmation of the diagnosis of the major sickling disorders, namely sickle-cell anaemia, Hb-SC disease, Hb-S/β-thal, and sickle-cell interacting with other haemoglobins. It must be emphasised at the outset that for accurate diagnosis, full consideration must be given to both the clinical and laboratory data. In some cases, it may be necessary to supplement these with family studies.

Sample collection and preparation
Sufficient sample for analysis can be obtained by finger or heel prick using ethylenediamine tetracetic acid (EDTA) as anticoagulant. (Samples collected into heparin may also be used but are not suitable for the preparation of blood films for the morphological analysis of the cells.) If refrigerated at 4°C, EDTA samples can still be used for electrophoresis for up to 28 to 30 days, but morphological analysis is best done as soon as possible after sample collection.

The haemogram
The initial clinical laboratory examination in any case suspected of sickle-cell disease, as in any other form of anaemia, is the haemogram or complete blood count. The aim is to describe the concentration of haemoglobin, and the number, size and volume of the erythrocytes as well as their individual content of haemoglobin. These tests are best performed with an electronic cell counter, but in the absence of such equipment, the measurement of the concen-

tration of haemoglobin and/or the packed cell volume (PCV) on a microhaematrocrit centrifuge, with the calculation of the mean corpuscular haemoglobin concentration (MCHC), are sufficient in the majority of cases. In sickle-cell anaemia, the anaemia is usually severe or moderately so (see Tables 5.4 and 6.1).

The stained blood smear (either Leishman or other Romanowsky stain) will show the morphology of the cells. The red cells are typically normocytic and normochromic, although some poikilocytosis and anisocytosis can often be seen. Target cells are common, and sickle-cell forms are characteristically found. Polychromasia, due to increased numbers of reticulocytes as a result of increased bone marrow activity, is also a constant feature, except on occasions of aplastic crises. Immature nucleated red cells may also be present. The findings in the various sickle-cell disease syndromes are compared in the Table 3.1.

Examination of the peripheral blood film may also be helpful in the diagnosis of some of the complications of sickle-cell disease. A raised peripheral blood white cell count, with a predominance of neutrophils, possibly showing immature forms and toxic granulation, is evidence of active infection. Malaria may be diagnosed by observing the parasites within the red cells, or by the presence of malarial pigment in the monocytes: malarial pigment is seen as brown lumps of varying size which take up no stain. If there are many (more than five per cent) neutrophils with five or more lobes to the nucleus, or nucleated red cells showing megaloblastic change, the patient is deficient in folic acid. Numerous platelets on the peripheral blood film suggest that the patient has had a recent infarctive crisis.

Haemoglobin electrophoresis

After the initial blood film examination, haemoglobin electrophoresis should be performed. This technique separates proteins on the basis of their electrical charge when in solution. The rate of migration of a protein in an electrical field is dependent not only on the charge, but also its size and structure, the pH and ionic strength of the buffer, the type of supporting medium used and the voltage applied. By altering these variables, several methods are now available for the separation and identification of haemoglobins.

Cellulose acetate membrane electrophoresis. For the diagnosis of sickle-cell disease, cellulose acetate membrane and paper are the commonest supporting media used for the initial electrophoretic analysis in alkaline buffers. Paper has the advantage of being simple and cheap, but it requires a longer time to separate. Furth-

Table 3.1 Laboratory findings in some common sickling disorders[a]

Disorder	Anaemia	Peripheral blood film	Cellulose acetate	Electrophoretic findings			
				Hb-F %	Hb-A$_2$ %	Hb-A %	HbS %
Sickle-cell trait (Hb-AS)	None	Normal	A + S	Normal	2·0–3·5	55–70	30–45
Sickle-cell anaemia (Hb-SS)	Severe	Sickle-cell forms, target cells, polychromasia, moderate anisopoikilocytosis	S(+F)	1–20	2·0–4·0	0	75–95
Sickle-cell-haemoglobin C disease (Hb-SC)	Mild to moderate	Target cells, mild anisopoikilocytosis	S + C	1–5	45–55[b] (C+A$_2$)	0	45–55
Sickle-cell-β-thalassaemia Hb-S/β$^+$thal	Moderate to severe	Microcytosis, target cells, hypochromia, marked anisopoikilocytosis, sickle-cell forms, nucleated red cells	S+F+A	2–10	4–8	10–30	60–85
Hb-S/β°thal			S + F	5–30	4–8	0	70–90
Sickle-cell-hereditary persistence of fetal haemoglobin (Hb-S/HPFH)	None to mild	Moderate anisocytosis, occasional target cells	S + F	15–35[c]	1·5–3·0	0	60–90
Sickle-cell-haemoglobin D disease (Hb-SD)	Mild to moderate	Anisopoikilocytosis, target cells	S[d]	1–5	2·0–3·5	0	95–99[d] (S+D)

[a] The sickling test is positive in all these syndromes.
[b] Hb-A$_2$ and Hb-C migrate together under the usual conditions for quantitating the haemoglobins.
[c] The cellular distribution of Hb-F is homogeneous. In all other conditions it is heterogeneous.
[d] Hb-S and Hb-D migrate together in alkaline buffers. They are clearly separated on citrate agar gel at acid pH.

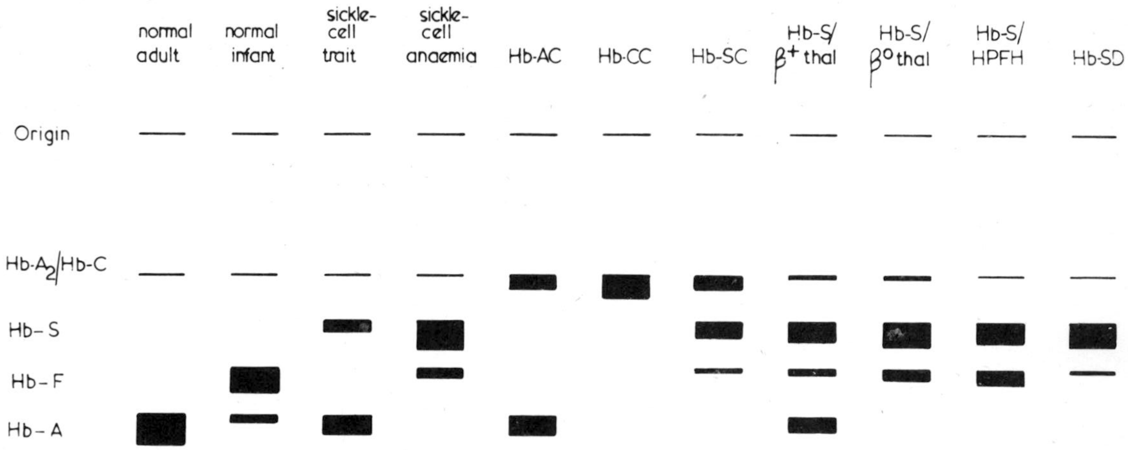

Fig. 3.1 Diagrammatic representation of haemoglobin electrophoretic patterns on cellulose acetate membrane.

ermore, absorption is considerable, making the elution and quantitation from such eluates of the separated haemoglobins impossible. Cellulose acetate, on the other hand, requires a much shorter period of electrophoresis, absorbs the haemoglobin only minimally and can be adapted for use when very small volumes of blood are available. This makes it especially suitable for screening purposes and it is the recommended method. The haemoglobins are identified by their position on the electrophoretogram. For example, Hb-A$_2$ and Hb-C move slowly and are closest to the origin; Hb-S, Hb-F and Hb-A move faster and are further from the origin in that order (Fig. 3.1). Hb-Barts, Hb-H and Hb-I move faster than Hb-A. It is useful to include a sample of known haemoglobin pattern when a run is made. This can be prepared from a patient with Hb-SC disease, or a composite mixture containing Hb-A,S,C and F can be specially prepared from blood samples with these haemoglobins.

The final identification of Hb-S cannot be said to have been completed with electrophoresis, because other haemoglobins, though less common, appear in the same position as Hb-S on electrophoresis in alkaline buffers. These include Hb-D and Hb-G-Philadelphia. In most instances, the Hb-S solubility test will confirm that the abnormal haemoglobin is in fact Hb-S, but if this test gives a negative result, electrophoresis on citrate agar will be necessary.

Citrate agar electrophoresis. Although a little more difficult and time-consuming than cellulose acetate, electrophoresis in citrate agar at acid pH 6·1 has the advantage of clearly differentiating between Hb-F,A,S and C, thus making the method the procedure of choice in screening cord bloods or samples from young infants. Hb-D also separates clearly from Hb-S in this system, migrating with Hb-A.

The sickling test
The sickling test is based on the fact that when red cells containing sickle haemoglobin are exposed to reduced oxygen tension, they assume the characteristic sickle shape. A drop of blood on a microscope slide is mixed with two drops of freshly prepared 2 per cent sodium metabisulphite. The preparation is covered with a coverslip which is sealed witth petroleum jelly to prevent drying, and examined under the microscope after 15 minutes, one hour and 24 hours. Cells containing 15 per cent or more Hb-S will sickle; this test does not distinguish between homozygotes and heterozygotes. False positive results may be obtained when poikilocytes are con-

fused with sickle-cell forms or when using a sodium metabisulphite solution which is greater than 2 per cent. False negative results are usually due to stale metabisulphite solution. They also occur frequently in the neonatal period because the proportion of Hb-S is below that required to deform the cells.

Solubility test

In the deoxygenated state, haemoglobin-S is much less soluble than normal haemoglobin. This property has been used as the basis of several tests, some of which are now available as commercial kits. Although the end point of solubility tests is clearer than that of sickling tests, the kits suffer from the same disability of not distinguishing clearly between the heterozygote and the homozygote. The 'test kits' also tend to be expensive. A recommended method is included in Appendix II; this is inexpensive and distinguishes homozygous sickle-cell anaemia from sickle-cell trait. It has the disadvantage of not distinguishing sickle-cell trait from doubly heterozygous forms of sickle-cell disease (Hb-SC etc.). The method has a place in outstation laboratories where haemoglobin electrophoresis is not available (Table 3.2), or where a result is required quickly, for example in the paediatric emergency ward or the anaesthetic room.

Table 3.2 Proposed choice of laboratory investigations for sickle-cell disease in hospitals in the tropics

Outstation or small hospital laboratories, paediatric emergency ward, anaesthetic room

    Haemoglobin concentration
    Peripheral blood film examination
    Hb-S solubility test

Hospitals with 100 or more beds

    As above, plus
    Packed cell volume (PCV) and mean corpuscular haemoglobin concentration
      (MCHC)
    Cellulose acetate membrane electrophoresis
    Alkali denaturation for Hb-F quantitation

Referral hospitals

    As above plus
    Citrate agar electrophoresis
    Hb-A_2 quantitation
    Kleihauer and Betke test for Hb-F-containing red cells
    Red cell indices by electronic cell counter

In centres where haemoglobin electrophoresis is readily available, the solubility test finds its greater use after, not before, electrophoresis has been completed. Samples that show a pattern migrating like Hb-S are subjected to the solubility test. This permits the simple detection of other abnormal haemoglobins, which, though migrating with Hb-S, will show normal solubility.

Haemoglobin-A_2 quantitation

Determination of the proportion of the total haemoglobin which is Hb-A_2 is an important diagnostic test when β-thal trait is suspected. Patients with β-thal trait usually have Hb-A_2 raised above 4 per cent. The haemoglobins are first separated by electrophoresis on cellulose acetate membrane. The portions containing the various fractions are cut out and eluted into small volumes of buffer. By comparing the optical densities at 415 nm, the relative proportions can be determined. This method has the disadvantage that it cannot be used in the presence of Hb-C, which migrates with Hb-A_2 (see Fig. 3.1). A microchromatographic method of using either DEAE sephadex or DEAE cellulose is also available and is suitable for screening large numbers.

Haemoglobin-F

The quantitation of fetal haemoglobin is based on its known property of resistance to denaturation by alkali. The one-minute alkali denaturation test of Singer or the two-minute denaturation test of Betke are the common methods used. The former is more accurate with larger amounts of Hb-F, while the latter is more acceptable with lower amounts.

The presence of red cells containing Hb-F can be detected by the elution technique of Kleihauer and Betke which depends on the observation that normal adult haemoglobin and other variants are soluble in citric acid phosphate buffer pH 3·3, whereas fetal haemoglobin is not. Cells containing Hb-F appear red, whereas cells not containing Hb-F show as ghosts after counterstaining with haematoxylin.

The proportion of Hb-F found in the 'Negro' type of hereditary persistence of fetal haemoglobin (HPFH) is generally higher than that found in subjects with sickle-cell anaemia. More than this, however, the cellular distribution of fetal haemoglobin is important, being homogeneous (equally distributed in all red cells) in HPFH and heterogeneous in sickle-cell anaemia and other situations.

Haemoglobin-G-Philadelphia

The α chain abnormality Hb-G-Philadelphia occurs in much less than 1 per cent of the population of West Africa, but it is the third commonest abnormal haemoglobin after Hb-S and Hb-C, and not infrequently leads to confusion in diagnosis.

The subject with Hb-AA plus Hb-G is clinically and haematologically normal, except for a band of Hb-G moving electrophoretically in the position of Hb-S. The Hb-S solubility test shows no precipitated Hb-S.

The subject with Hb-AS plus Hb-G is also clinically and haematologically normal. Haemoglobin electrophoresis on cellulose acetate reveals three major bands in the position of Hb-A, Hb-S and Hb-C. The patient has in fact four major haemoglobins: (i) Hb-A, (ii) Hb-S, (iii) Hb-G moving with Hb-S and (iv) the hybrid Hb-S/G ($\alpha_2^G \beta_2^S$), which moves in the position of Hb-C.

The subject with Hb-SS plus Hb-G shows all the clinical and haematological features of sickle-cell disease. Haemoglobin electrophoresis on cellulose acetate shows a pattern similar to Hb-SC, due to the presence of two haemoglobins, Hb-S and Hb-S/G, in the position of Hb-C. The patient is likely to be diagnosed as having Hb-SC disease, but the blood picture and the severity of the disease point against this. If the haemoglobin-S solubility test is performed, both haemoglobins are precipitated to give a pattern like Hb-SS, so demonstrating easily that the patient does not have Hb-SC disease.

In any of these three situations, or others where results are confusing, the patients, or the specimens of blood, should be referred to a specialist haematology department.

SUMMARY

The laboratory diagnosis of sickle-cell disease is simple and relatively inexpensive: doctors should insist on certain tests being available wherever the sickle gene is prevalent. At the simplest level, accurate laboratory diagnosis may be made in most patients with only the haemoglobin concentration, peripheral blood film examination and the Hb-S solubility test (see Table 3.2). It is reasonable to insist that in a laboratory of a hospital with 100 beds or more cellulose acetate membrane electrophoresis should be available: the diagnosis of sickle-cell anaemia can be made with certainty in the majority of patients when the clinical picture, the blood film and the haemoglobin electrophoretic pattern are typical, and all the haemoglobin is precipitated in the Hb-S solubility test. When there is a difficulty in diagnosis, further tests should be performed, probably in a referral or specialist hospital (see Table 3.2).

REFERENCES

Dacie, J.V. & Lewis, S.M. (1975) *Practical Haematology*, 5th edn., Ch. 10. Edinburgh: Churchill Livingstone.

Efremor, G.D. & Huisman, T.H.J. (1974) The laboratory diagnosis of haemoglobinopathies. *Clinics in Haematology*,3, 527–570.

Lehmann, H. & Huntsman, R.G. (1975) *Laboratory detection of haemoglobinopathies.* Association of Clinical Pathologists, Broadsheet 33.

Schmidt, R.M. & Brosious, E.M. (1976) *Basic Laboratory Methods of Hemoglobinopathy Detection*, 6th edn. US Department of Health, Education and Welfare Publication No. CDC 76-8266.

Schneider, R.G. (1978) Methods for detection of hemoglobinopathies in the routine clinical laboratory. *CRC Critical Reviews in Clinical Laboratory Sciences*, **9**, 243–271.

The pathology of sickle-cell disease

Sickling in the body is a capillary phenomenon. Deoxygenation of haemoglobin takes place in tissue capillaries, with alteration of the physico-chemical structure of the abnormal Hb-S molecule resulting in deformation of the red cells to the abnormal sickle shape. This process is not initiated in the aorta, arteries or the heart because of the high oxygen tension in these locations. Even during crisis, when there is massive sickling, the process is restricted to those parts of the cardiovascular system where deoxygenation takes place. Sickling is a continuing process in the patient with sickle-cell anaemia. In Hb-SC disease, and other sickle-cell diseases, it is usually intermittent, as there is a sufficiently high proportion of the other, non-sickling, haemoglobin to prevent continuous sickling of the Hb-S. However, in times of stress, sickling occurs as an episodic phenomenon producing clinical crises. Crises are more common and more severe in Hb-SS patients than in the double heterozygotes.

Many of the clinical manifestations and pathological aspects of sickle-cell anaemia and other sickle-cell diseases are related to the effects of the sickling phenomenon. It is possible, however, that other factors so far not properly or fully identified contribute to the morbidity and mortality in sickle-cell disease.

Basic pathology
The outstanding primary effects of sickling are (i) those of intracapillary sludging of the deformed red cells, and (ii) chronic haemolytic anaemia resulting from removal of the deformed (sickled) red cells. There is also evidence of decreased immune competence in the patient.

Red cell sludging and infarction
The effects of intracapillary aggregation of red cells are (i) stasis with its intravascular complications, and (ii) the consequences of tissue anoxia. Intracapillary red cell sludging and resultant stasis

produce capillary endothelial anoxic damage. Under these conditions, thrombosis occurs in the capillaries. In the process of thrombosis, there is consumption of platelets and some coagulation factors so that these are decreased in the blood. The breakdown of thrombi results in increased amounts of fibrin degradation products (FDP) in circulation. Damage to the endothelium of capillaries also leads to exudation of plasma into the surrounding soft tissues, contributing to soft tissue swellings classically seen in dactylitis and the hand-foot syndrome. The tissues suffer anoxia, the severity of which depends on the collateral capillary circulation. The combination of ischaemia and oedema stimulates the nerve endings in tissues to produce pain, which may be severe. The most serious effect of tissue ischaemia is infarction (Fig. 4.1).

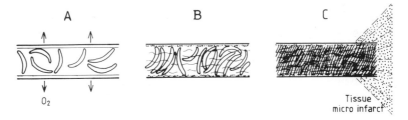

Fig. 4.1 Effects of deoxygenation in tissue capillaries: A. Sickling of erythrocytes, B. Sludging, stasis, anoxic endothelial damage, C. Thrombosis and microinfarct.

The infarct, being induced by capillary blockage, is a microinfarct. In the early stages, the infarct may be haemorrhagic depending upon the looseness of the tissue. Thus, marrow and splenic infarcts are haemorrhagic while bone infarcts are not. Coalescence of these microinfarcts may produce relatively large infarcts which by their nature present irregular outlines. They do not present the sharply demarcated conical or triangular outlines of arterial infarcts. Infarcts may occur in any tissue, and their effects in the different organs will be described later in a systematic order. Healing of infarcts is by scarring which leaves primarily a microscopic scar but may be extensive if the infarct is a large coalesced one.

Haemolysis
Anaemia is a constant feature in sickle-cell anaemia (Hb-SS). The organs are pale, the degree of pallor depending upon the severity of the anaemia. Patients who die in haemolytic crisis may present with dramatically low PCV (for example, PCV 0·06) during their terminal crisis.

Haemolytic hyperbilirubinaemia, usually with clinical jaundice, is a constant feature in sickle-cell anaemia and a common feature in other sickle-cell diseases during crisis, the depth of icterus depending upon the severity of haemolysis. The hyperbilirubinaemia conveys an icteric tinge to organs in addition to the pallor of anaemia.

In the presence of continuous or episodic haemolysis, the iron which is liberated from haemolysed red cells is stored in the internal organs and the marrow. As the body does not have an efficient system for disposing of iron, haemosiderosis of some degree is a constant features in sickle-cell anaemia and frequent in other sickle-cell diseases. It is unusual for tissues to react to the iron excess by fibrosis, although this has occasionally been encountered. Patients with sickle-cell disease should not be treated with oral or parenteral iron, as this adds to the excessive deposition of the iron in the tissues. Repeated transfusions with blood or packed red cells also lead to haemosiderosis. In the presence of haemosiderosis, the organs and tissues take on a brown hue.

Infection and resistance of infection
Persons with sickle-cell disease are abnormally susceptible to bacterial infections, especially those under the age of seven years. The course of infection tends to be severe, and complicated by anaemia and infarctive crises. Infections are frequently the direct or contributory causes of death, especially in early childhood.

The most common of these severe infections are pneumonia, meningitis, general sepsis, osteomyelitis and pyelonephritis. The frequency of invasion by different organisms reflects both the susceptibility of the host and the prevalence of the organisms in the environment. Pneumonia is commonly caused by *Diplococcus pneumoniae, Salmonella* (especially in Africa) and mycoplasma. The organisms of meningitis are commonly *D. pneumoniae* or *Haemophilus influenzae*; in the savanna areas of Africa there are seasonal epidemics of meningococcal meningitis, and the patients with sickle-cell disease are more susceptible than the rest of the population. The infecting organisms of generalised septicaemia are frequently the same as those causing pneumonia, meningitis or osteomyelitis.

The pus from osteomyelitis often yields more than one organism, and the bacteria isolated in one Nigerian series included Salmonella (45 per cent), coliforms (45 per cent), *Staphlococcus pyogenes* (20 per cent), and *Staph. epidermidis*, Klebsiella and pseudomonas (7·5 per cent). Salmonella infections appear to be becoming less common in America, where pneumococcal osteomyelitis is reported. The organisms isolated from patients with bacteriuria include *E. coli*, coliforms, and Klebsiella.

There is some evidence of an increased incidence of tuberculosis as a cause of death among patients with sickle-cell disease in Africa, but not in America.

Acute viral infections are more severe than in the rest of the population and are frequent precipitants of infarctive crises (Powars, 1975); bulbar poliomyelitis has been described as a cause of death.

The impairment of resistance to infection in sickle-cell disease has several different mechanisms (Barrett-Connor, 1971; Powars, 1975; Hand and King, 1978).

1. There is a defect of the alternative pathway of complement activation and opsonisation, contributing to increased susceptibility to pneumococcus and Salmonella..

2. Neutrophil and macrophage activity is impaired.

3. There is functional hyposplenism, further decreasing macrophage function and immune responses to organisms in the blood.

4. Haemolysis increases susceptibility to Salmonella and other organisms, possibly by making iron available for bacterial metabolism.

5. Postinfarctive tissue necrosis precedes the development of osteomyelitis and pyelonephritis; the frequency of these two complications remains high after childhood, being dependent on tissue necrosis rather than the immature immune state; pyelonephritis is particularly frequent during pregnancy.

6. There is some evidence of diminished cell-mediated immunity, which could contribute to the susceptibility to viral infections. Humoral immunity is unimpaired, and immunoglobulin (Ig)M levels tend to be high in response to frequent infections.

Hb-SS subjects have partial protection against *P. falciparum* (like Hb-AS) and *P. malariae* (unlike Hb-AS); however, malaria, even if less intense than in normal persons, has grave consequences; it is a frequent trigger to haemolytic and infarctive crises and is a common cause of death in sickle-cell anaemia (Molineaux *et al.*, 1979).

Crisis
Factors responsible for the variation of the type of crisis are not clear, and frequently a combination of crisis types is seen. Thrombotic or infarctive crises are often accompanied by haemolysis.

Anaemic crises. A rapid worsening of anaemia may be due to (i) haemolytic crisis, (ii) sequestration crisis, (iii) aplastic (or hypoplastic) crisis, or (iv) acute megaloblastic arrest of erythropoiesis.

Rapid haemolysis (without enlargement of the spleen) is a common complication of viral, bacterial or protozoal (malarial) infection. Similar infective causes can alter the red cell membrane and so lead to acute sequestration in the spleen. The spleen enlarges dramatically and the PCV falls precipitately. Sequestration crises are encountered most frequently in Hb-SC disease in pregnancy, although they may occur in other patients, including children with Hb-SS.

Aplastic or marrow-suppressive crises are the least frequently encountered by pathologists, and are related to septicaemia.

Folate deficiency has a multiple aetiology in sickle-cell disease. There is anorexia, possibly malabsorption, and a greatly increased requirement for folate to meet the demand of erythroid hyperplasia. The already embarrassed folate status may be precipitated into acute megaloblastic arrest of erythropoiesis through the inactivation of the enzyme dihydrofolate reductase by pyrexia of infection.

Infarctive crisis. Acute severe pain as a mode of presentation is relatively common and is due to tissue infarcts. This is most frequently skeletal. Internal organ pain presenting as acute abdominal or less frequently as severe chest pain is caused by organ infarction. The commonest is abdominal or left hypochondrial pain due to splenic infarcts. Other tissues may suffer infarcts, or there may be referred infarctive pain, the source of which the surgeon may fail to identify at laparotomy. In such cases, it is common to presume appendiceal pain and perform appendicectomy. The specimen usually presents no evidence of active inflammation and it is common for the pathologist to suggest the correct diagnosis by identifying massive sickling of red cells in the blood vessels of the appendix.

Investigation of the patient in crisis. Although all sickling crises must be treated with special care, it seems that some factors or signs have a sinister connotation. Very low PCV and high blood levels of bilirubin indicate severe haemolysis. Where facilities are available for such investigations, reduced platelet counts and low activity of coagulation factors with high levels of FDP indicate extensive capillary thrombosis. There is a rebound thrombocytosis (obvious on a blood film) and a raised fibrinogen concentration during recovery.

Attention has been drawn to pyrexia during crisis as a sinister factor (Attah, 1975). Most sickle-cell disease deaths are associated with pyrexia during the fatal crisis. In some of these, there is a concomitant or complicating condition which may produce fever, but in a large number of patients, no such condition is present and the fever is probably due to body reaction to infarcted tissue. In such cases, the temperature is usually less than 38·3°C. In the majority, the peripheral blood white cell count is in the normal

range, but a few have a leucocytosis with a slight neutrophil predominance.

Growth

The growth and general development of the child with sickle-cell
anaemia is usually retarded, while with other sickle-cell diseases it is
normal. However, retardation of growth in sickle-cell anaemia
seems to be influenced by the environment. In children with lower
than average body weight, organ weights are also low. There is no
abnormality of functional development of organs.

Factors affecting the severity of sickle-cell disease

The severity of sickle-cell anaemia is variable, and both environmental and genetic factors affect the prognosis (Table 4.1). In Africa, the environmental factors are certainly, the more important,
but the genetic factors have become more obvious where better
standards of hygiene and nutrition have been achieved.

Table 4.1 Factors improving the prognosis and survival of patients with sickle-cell
anaemia

Environmental	Genetic
Parents — intelligent	High Hb-F
— careful	α-thalassaemia
— well educated	Unknown genetic factors?
— of good economic state	
Protection against or absence of malaria	
Good hygiene	
Good nutrition	
Accessible medical care	

The environment. The severity of sickle-cell disease in a community is an expression of the background of health in that community.
Sickling crises are precipitated by raised temperature, bacteriuria,
infection with other invading organisms, acidosis and dehydration.
The clinical translation of these factors in the African environment is either malaria (Konotey-Ahulu, 1971) or bacterial infections (Attah and Ekere, 1975). There is no doubt that the poorly
nourished among these children fare worse when challenged by
these infections. In the rural African community, where hygiene
and nutrition are poor and where antimalarial prophylactics. mos-
quito avoidance and modern medicine are unknown, about 95 per
cent of all children born with sickle-cell anaemia die before the age
of five years (Molineaux et al., 1979). Those who survive show advanced tissue and organ alteration by the age of puberty.

On the other hand, infants and children with sickle-cell disease whose parents are intelligent, careful, educated and relatively well-to-do in the developing countries, and patients living in advanced countries, may suffer little morbidity and live to relatively advanced age. Factors which contribute to this wellbeing include the absence of malaria, high standards of hygiene, good nutrition and adequate medical supervision, including obstetric care.

Haemoglobin-F concentration. In the majority of Hb-SS persons, the proportion of haemoglobin which is Hb-F is more than 1 per cent after infancy. There is both a persisting high rate of synthesis and a preferential survival of red cells containing a high concentration of Hb-F, which is distributed unevenly between the red cells, as shown by the acid elution test.

The mean proportion of Hb-F in Africans with Hb-SS is about 5 per cent in males and 6 per cent in females; few have more than 10 per cent, but the occasional patient may have up to 30 per cent (Serjeant, 1975). In Hb-SS persons in Arabia, Iran and India, the mean proportion of Hb-F is about 20 per cent, with a range of 8 to 36 per cent (Huisman, 1979). The cause of the raised Hb-F levels in the occasional Negro patient and in these Asian populations is not completely understood.

Hb-F does not participate with Hb-S in gel formation and it has a high oxygen affinity. These two properties tend to prevent sickling by dilution of Hb-S and by maintaining a high oxygen saturation within the red cell. A high proportion of Hb-F in sickle-cell anaemia is associated with a more normal red cell morphology, fewer irreversibly sickled cells in the peripheral blood, longer red cell survival, less blood vessel obstruction, less infarction, less splenic atrophy, less bodily abnormality, a more normal rate of growth and development, and a generally milder expression of the disease.

α-*Thalassaemia.* The diagnosis of α-thalassaemia is difficult except in the newborn, and estimates of gene frequencies in Negro populations have ranged from 2 to 30 per cent. The gene in Negroes is that for α-thalassaemia 2 (-α) so that the possible expressions are heterozygous (-α/α α) and homozygous (-α/-α).

The associated inheritance of homozygous α thalassaemia 2 (-α/-α) with homozygous sickle-cell anaemia (β^S/β^S) results in a mild clinical and haematological expression of sickle-cell anaemia, probably because the rates of synthesis of α chains and β chains are balanced. The heterozygous inheritance of α-thalassaemia 2 with sickle-cell anaemia (-α/α α: β^s/β^s) has no apparent effect on the severity of sickle-cell anaemia, and this may account for the widely differing expression of Hb-SS, even within the same family.

It should be remembered that the diagnosis of Hb-SS may be incorrect in some patients with few complications; possible diagnoses include Hb-SD-Ibadan, Hb-S/β °thal and Hb-S/HPHF (see Ch. 3).

Systemic review

Bones and bone marrow

The bone marrow, in response to continuous or episodic intense haemolysis, is hyperplastic. The marrow is consequently red marrow, even in adult patients, and displays lines of expansion into the compact cortical portions of long bones. Marrow space in cancellous bones is also expanded. Along with this, marrow infarcts occur during crises, which may be restricted or extensive. They are haemorrhagic in the early stage, changing to yellow and becoming sclerosed with healing and reconstituting marrow in time. The best area to demonstrate these alterations is in the marrow of long bones, for instance the femur. Recent marrow infarct fragments may break into marrow veins, as the infarct is loose and friable. These result in marrow embolism to the lungs which may be diagnosed by staining the sputum with Sudan red and so demonstrating fat globules.

Alterations in the bones themselves are easily demonstrated on X-ray. These are an interplay between marrow expansion in the bone and bone infarcts with sclerosis. Infarcts in bones are common and contribute to skeletal pain in crises along with marrow infarcts. The periosteum is often involved, and periosteal reaction is frequently seen on X-ray and contributes to the hand-foot syndrome. The bones of the skull, especially the calvarium (the thickness of which is normally mostly constituted by marrow-rich diploe), become markedly expanded. This is responsible for clinical bossing of the head. It also conveys characteristic, though not diagnostic, radiological appearances, the most widely recognised pattern being the hair-on-end appearance. Curvilinear stripes are perhaps equally common. In the long bones, the marrow lines in the cortex are fancifully compared to railway lines and are described as 'rail roading' (see Ch. 8). Chronic osteomyelitis is relatively frequent in these patients. Avascular necrosis of the head and neck of femur and of other bones may be seen in older patients.

Cardiovascular system

The heart displays alterations of chronic anaemic disease and is usually slightly enlarged in patients with sickle-cell anaemia. In those with severe anaemia, and in crises, cardiac decompensation may occur and the patients present in frank cardiac failure. In these cases, cardiomegaly may be marked. The epicardium is usually smooth and the myocardium is pale. There is hypertrophy of the left ventricular wall and dilatation of all chambers. No abnormalities of the valves are present. The coronary arteries are not remarkable although there is evidence of occlusive abnormalities in their microcirculation. The aorta and major blood vessels show no abnormalities.

Pulmonary system

In the respiratory tract, changes directly due to sickle-cell disease are limited to congestion in the majority of cases. Bone marrow emboli in the smaller branches of pulmonary arteries are present in a proportion of cases. In a minority of these, they probably contribute to demise or pose a serious clinical problem. It is unusual for them to cause pulmonary infarcts. Pulmonary infarction due to sludging of sickled erythrocytes is uncommon because of the dual blood supply to the lungs and the fact that almost all pulmonary capillaries are in near-direct contact with inspired oxygen-rich air in the alveoli. However, pulmonary infarcts do occur, and their cumulative effect leads to interstitial fibrosis in adult life. Pneumonia is common at autopsy. Massive pulmonary haemorrhage and haemorrhagic pleural effusions are uncommon findings at autopsy, and are probably terminal events.

Gastrointestinal system

In the gastrointestinal tract, the mucosa is pale and may be oedematous. No specific or frequently associated lesions have been identified, but, rarely haemorrhagic peritoneal effusions are found at autopsy.

The liver capsule is smooth and is usually moderately enlarged. There is variable congestion. The liver substance may be pale as a result of anaemia, yellow and fatty in malnourished patients, or present a brown hue in those with haemosiderosis. Hepatic infarcts have been described occasionally; their rarity is, again, probably a result of a double blood supply and the fact that blood perfuses hepatocytes through sinusoids which practically encircle liver cell cords on all surfaces. When cirrhosis occurs in a patient with sickle-cell disease, it is most likely caused by factors in the environment other than sickle-cell disease itself, although excess iron pigment may perhaps be a contributory factor.

In the presence of continuous or episodic severe haemolysis, it would be expected that patients with sickle-cell disease develop pigment gallstones. The development of gallstones, however, seems to be influenced by dietary environmental factors. Consequently, although pigment stones are common in American children with sickle-cell disease, they are currently uncommon in African patients.

The spleen

Changes in the spleen attract considerable attention because of the clinical frequency of infarcts and splenomegaly in younger patients, and markedly shrunken spleens at autopsy in older patients with sickle-cell anaemia. The spleen continuously removes from the circulation and destroys the large numbers of sickled and fragmented red cells, and so is congested and enlarged in young children. Infarcts, which may occur during crises or between crises, are minute initially but coalesce to form relatively large infarcts. An unusual manifestation is infarction of the whole spleen. The infarcts are haemorrhagic owing to the loose structure of the spleen. Reaction to infarction is congestion in the rest of the spleen. The result of this is further enlargement of the spleen, sometimes markedly so, in children with sickle-cell disease. The spleen remains enlarged into adult life only in those patients with milder forms of sickle-cell disease, in those with high Hb-F or those who are well nourished, have protection against malaria and other infections, and receive adequate medical attention.

In most patients with sickle-cell anaemia, repeated frequent infarcts result in healing by scarring and fibrotic contraction of the spleen. Thus, the spleen which is enlarged and congested in the infant and child becomes gradually scarred and permanently contracted by the age of puberty in most African children with sickle-cell anaemia. This process is commonly referred to as autosplenectomy. The splenic scars contain iron from the breakdown of red cells and are referred to as fibrosiderotic nodules. The older scars may become calcified. The capsule of the spleen is fibrosed and irregularly thickened as a result of infarcts or exudative fibrinous reactions. This may result in adhesions to the peritoneum and surrounding organs.

Another feature of the spleen which is of interest is the development of pulp nodules in the splenic substance. These protrude as elevations from the cut surface of the spleen between the scarred

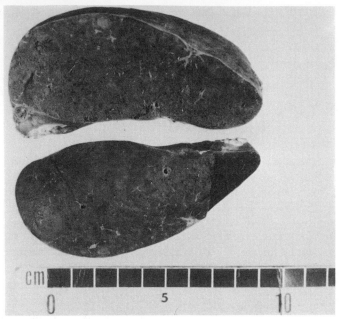

Fig. 4.2 Scarred contracted spleen with pulp regeneration nodules.

contracted tissue (Fig. 4.2). Their development is probably a consequence of the need for an active spleen to combat endemic diseases, such as malaria. In some patients, prominent accessory spleens are present.

Genitourinary system
Hyposthenuria as a renal functional disorder is a constant feature of sickle-cell anaemia, and chronic pyelonephritis is common. The kidneys may be of normal size or slightly contracted. The capsules are variably adherent and the renal surfaces may display irregular shallow scars of chronic pyelonephritis. In some cases, however, these changes may be minimal or not obvious. Cut surfaces of the kidneys reveal congestion with a background of pale renal substance. The cortex and medulla usually retain their normal thickness proportions. There is blunting of the renal papillae in cases of established chronic pyelonephritis. Microscopy confirms these findings, including interstitial chronic inflammatory infiltrates in chronic pyelonephritis.

A feature of interest is the appearance in some cases of telangiectatic dilated capillaries in the medulla. The most prominent of these lesions have been described as 'capillary lakes' in an adult male with Hb-SC disease. It is likely that these or related lesions are responsible for the haematuria which is a clinical problem in sickle-cell haemoglobinopathy. They represent exaggerated compensatory capillary dilatation following medullary capillary bed thrombosis and scarring. Microscopic haematuria is relatively common in sickle-cell disease, and frank haematuria is sometimes a serious intractable clinical problem. Nephrectomy has been performed on patients in whom it was not otherwise possible to control unilateral haematuria. Great care must be exercised in selecting patients for nephrectomy, as the other kidney may subsequently develop haematuria. This problem is most common among Hb-SC patients and, curiously, is next most frequently seen among Hb-AS individuals (see Ch. 2). Hb-SS patients show this complication the least, but it is not clear if this is related to the young age of the majority of Hb-SS patients.

Some sickle-cell patients present with nephrotic syndrome. It must be borne in mind in such instances that a patient with sickle-cell disease may acquire nephrotic syndrome as the result of one of the usual causes of this syndrome, including drugs, cardiovascular causes, metabolic disorders (e.g. amyloidosis and diabetes mellitus) and all forms of glomerulonephritis. It is therefore essential to investigate the patient fully to exclude these causes before presuming sickle-cell disease as the primary cause of the syndrome. Such investigations include renal biopsy. Even with full histologic study, the question may remain unsettled, as lipoid nephrosis must be a differential diagnosis. In this condition, there may be no appreciable histologic abnormalities on light microscopy. Electron microscopy settles this problem. In nephrosis due to sickle-cell disease, the mechanism of causation is probably sludging of red cells in glomerular capillaries with stasis producing anoxic damage to the glomerular endothelium with consequent leakage of protein.

The ureters and urinary bladder are usually normal. The gonads may manifest delayed maturation, but there are no other abnormalities. Other sexual organs are unremarkable, except with the complication of priapism (see Ch. 6).

Central nervous system
Neurological symptoms are not infrequent and are due to ischaemia and microscopic infarcts of the brain and spinal cord. The brain is pale and the leptomeninges are variably congested. The cerebral substance is also congested with a pale background. Subarachnoid haemorrhages are only occasionally found at autopsy. Paraplegia is a rare complication, probably due to extensive microvascular damage to the spinal cord, or to cerebral haemorrhage.

The skin

Chronic ulcers of the skin are caused by dermal capillary thrombosis with skin infarction which — though small at first — may coalesce to form relatively large infarcts which ulcerate. They seem to be less common in African patients than in American blacks. As the microcirculation is damaged, these ulcers tend to be chronic and heal with difficulty. The most frequent location is in the lower extremities.

Death in sickle-cell anaemia

Death from sickle-cell anaemia is unusual in the first six months of life; there is a peak of mortality around the age of two years in both Africa (Molineaux et al., 1979) and America (Powars, 1975). Thereafter, up to the age of about seven years, morbidity and mortality decline gradually as immunity to infection is acquired. Surviving patients usually enjoy a period of relatively good health until about adult life. There are then the complications and deaths associated with pregnancy (see Ch. 7). Irreversible degeneration of organs (kidney, lungs, liver, heart, bones and joints) leads to increasing morbidity and mortality in both sexes from about 20 years in Africa and about 30 years in America.

The immediate causes of death in sickle-cell anaemia and sickle-cell disease are many. Severe infections in children with sickle-cell anaemia are common. These may be malarial or acute bacterial, and the most frequent of the latter are pneumonia, meningitis and septicaemia. Patients with sickle-cell anaemia seem to have a greater susceptibility to the bacterial infections than those with heterozygous sickle-cell disease (Attah and Ekere, 1975). Severe viral infections may also be present. The infections precipitate severe sickling in these patients. However, in about two thirds of patients there is no evidence of infection at autopsy, and death is probably directly due to crisis and sickle-cell disease per se. The precise mechanism of death is unclear in many such instances. In patients with such demonstrable phenomena as subarachnoid haemorrhage and massive pulmonary haemorrhage, the cause of death is obvious. In others, it is probably a combination of severe haemolytic anaemia, cardiac failure and extensive microvascular disease with damage to vital cerebral centres. There may be other as yet unelicited mechanisms of death.

Death in adults with Hb-SC disease is frequently not the result of the haemoglobinopathy. When due to the disease, it usually follows a crisis during periods of physiologic or pathologic stress. In women, death is most frequently related to pregnancy and child-

birth. In these patients, death may occur through one or a combination of the mechanisms already described. On the other hand,
some special phenomena associated with pregnancy or childbirth
may occur, for instance preeclamptic toxaemia or eclampsia. Severe
sequestration crises are frequent in pregnant patients, producing
massive pooling of blood in the spleen and circulatory failure.

Unexplained sudden death
Sudden deaths among children with sickle-cell anaemia are probably more common than is generally appreciated. Children may die
in their sleep without apparent crisis. Following such deaths, a
specimen of heart blood for haemoglobin electrophoresis may give
the diagnosis in a previously unknown patient if there has been no
recent blood transfusion. Post-mortem X-ray examination of bones,
especially the calvarium, demonstrates expanded diploe with the
characteristic appearances. Examination of long bones, especially
the femur, usually shows 'rail-roading' of the cortex by expanded
bone marrow and frequently bone marrow infarcts.

Case history 1. The patient was a four-year-old boy who suddenly
developed acute mental symptoms. He was taken to a hospital
casualty department, but his symptoms had subsided by the time
of arrival. A thorough examination demonstrated no central nervous system signs and the child appeared to be in good health. He
was observed for one hour and discharged home. The parents had
failed to give the doctor the information that this child was known
to have sickle-cell anaemia. Shortly after arriving home, the mental
symptoms reappeared and the patient was taken back to the hospital. He died on arrival.

Case history 2. Another sudden death occurred in a four-year-old
girl who had suffered several episodes of unexplained but trouble-
some illness apart from the usual childhood diseases, such as
measles. On each occasion the child had attended a university
medical centre and had been seen by doctors. Probably because she
was a well-developed, apparently healthy child, there was no suspicion or diagnosis of sickle-cell anaemia. During one such unexplained episode, the child died within three hours of the onset of
illness. Haemoglobin electrophoresis was performed on a blood
specimen which had been taken before death and this showed Hb-
SS.

Conclusion
About 95 per cent of Hb-SS children in rural Africa die before the
age of five years where there is no medical care (Molineaux *et al.*,

83922

1979). Up to two thirds die by the age of five years even when they attend hospitals in Africa (Attah and Ekere, 1975).

The pattern of pathologic manifestations and death in sickle-cell disease in Africa will change with the general improvement in population and environmental health. With wider availability of medical care, children will suffer fewer crises, will receive adequate care during crises and so survive into adult life. Organ changes will be delayed and perhaps be less severe.

REFERENCES

Attah, Ed. 'B. (1975) Malignant febrile crisis in sickle-cell anaemia. *East African Medical Journal*, 52, 467–469.

Attah, Ed. 'B. & Ekere, M.C. (1975) Death patterns in sickle cell anemia. *Journal of the American Medical Association*, 233, 889–890.

Barrett-Connor, E. (1971) Bacterial infection and sickle cell anemia. An analysis of 250 infections in 166 patients and a review of the literature. *Medicine*, 50, 97–112.

Hand, W.L. & King, N.L. (1978) Serum opsonization of Salmonella in sickle cell anemia. *American Journal of Medicine*, 64, 388–395.

Huisman, T.H.J. (1979) Sickle cell anemia as a syndrome: a review of diagnostic features. *American Journal of Hematology*, 6, 173–184.

Konotey-Ahulu, F.I.D. (1971) Malaria and sickle cell disease. *British Medical Journal*, 2, 710–711.

Molineaux, L., Fleming, A.F., Cornille-Brøgger, R., Kagan, I. & Storey, J. (1979) Abnormal haemoglobins in the Sudan savanna of Nigeria. III. Malaria, immunoglobulins and antimalarial antibodies in sickle cell disease. *Annals of Tropical Medicine and Parasitology*, 73, 301–310.

Powars D.R. (1975)'Natural history of sickle cell disease — the first ten years. *Seminars in Hematology*, 12, 267–235.

Serjeant, G.R. (1975) Fetal haemoglobin in homozygous sickle cell disease. *Clinics in Haematology*, 4, 109–122.

Sickle-cell disease in childhood

The number of patients with sickle-cell disease attending regularly at the Anaemia Clinic of the Children's Department of University College Hospital (UCH), Ibadan, Nigeria, has increased from 200 in 1959 (Hendrickse, 1960) to about 2500 in 1979; the total attendances are about 6000 per year (Table 5.1).

Table 5.1 Attendance at the Anaemia Clinic of the Children's Department, University College Hospital, Ibadan, Nigeria.

Year	New patients per year	Total attendance per year	Average attendance per clinic
1968–69	112	4287	84
1969–70	122	3588	69
1970–71	159	3457	68
1971–72	151	5599	115
1972–73	231	5753	127
1977–78	353	5922	118

Most patients with sickle-cell disease present in infancy and early childhood, and only in a small number is the condition mild enough to delay its manifestation until adolescence or early adult life. The majority of these patients have sickle-cell anaemia (Hb-SS), and the description which follows applies to this condition unless otherwise stated. Although sickle-cell anaemia is the more severe and a frequently fatal disease, children with Hb-SC disease present with almost all the features which are common in sickle-cell anaemia. There are, however, some complications which are more common in Hb-SC disease; these include ocular lesions and splenic infarct during air travel (see Ch. 6). Other sickle-cell diseases, such as Hb-S/β^+ thal, are rarer and generally much milder.

CLINICAL FEATURES

Common symptoms in infancy and childhood are fever, pain and swelling of the limbs, pain and swelling of the abdomen, poor appetite, vomiting and diarrhoea. The most characteristic symptoms are pain and swelling of the limbs and abdomen, and these are frequently confused with rheumatism and surgical abdomen respectively. Other common symptoms include epistaxis, bleeding gums, passage of dark urine, polyuria and polydypsia. Dark urine is due to haemolysis in most cases and only occasionally to haematuria.

Age at presentation

Before three months of age, the high level of Hb-F generally suppresses sickling. Presentation at this age is, therefore, unusual, although infection, haemolysis and jaundice, even in the newborn, have been described (anon., 1978). Of about 1800 Nigerian children, 0·3 per cent were aged between three and five months (Table 5.2). About 10 per cent were seen for the first time between six and twelve months, while 80 per cent were seen for the first time between 13 months and 10 years of age. It is also worth noting that about 10 per cent of these children presented when they were aged

Table 5.2   Age distribution of 1877 children with sickle-cell disease when first seen at University College Hospital, Ibadan, Nigeria.

Age	Number	% of total
< 3 months	—	—
3– 5 months	6	0·3
6– 9 months	25	1·3
10–12 months	156	8·3
13–36 months	617	32·9
4– 6 years	469	25·0
7–10 years	410	21·8
< 10 years	194	10·4
Total	1877	100

Table 5.3   Age at time of presentation of children with Hb-SS and Hb-SC disease at University College Hospital, Ibadan, Nigeria.

Age in years	Hb-SS % of total	Hb-SC % of total
< ½	6·2	6·5
½–2	45·5	39·8
>2–4	18·7	19·4
>4–6	13·2	15·0
>6–8	9·0	11·8
> 8	7·4	7·5

above 10 years, and a good proportion of them were diagnosed on routine haematological investigation. The age distribution at first attendance with Hb-SC disease is almost identical with that for patients with Hb-SS (Table 5.3).

Sickle-cell habitus

Certain characteristic physical appearances, referred to as the sickle-cell habitus, have been described in some patients, particularly those aged eight years and above. The limbs are thin and long, and the abdomen protuberant with exaggerated lumber lordosis. Height and weight are below average for the age. The head is frequently large and abnormally shaped as a result of bossing of frontal and parietal bones (Fig. 5.1). The maxilla is prominent with resultant

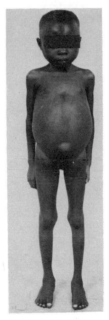

Fig. 5.1 Sickle-cell habitus in a 10-year-old girl.

depression of the bridge of the nose and protrusion of the upper teeth, which override the lower ones (gnathopathy). The chest is frequently barrel-shaped due to increase in the anteroposterior diameter. The eyes and lips reveal pallor and icterus. While these features are quite common and characteristic in some children, a large number of patients are well proportioned and robust.

Sickle-cell crises

Sickle-cell crises are among the most characteristic features of this disease. They are episodic attacks which come and go without warning. Factors known to precipitate crises include infections (malarial, bacterial and viral), cold and wet weather, starvation, exertion and any other conditions which may cause dehydration and acidosis. Thus, crises are more frequent when the cold wind, called the *harmattan*, blows off the Sahara desert, in the rainy season and particularly during seasonal changes. It is important that parents are told about these precipitating factors, so that extra precautions are taken not to expose their children unduly at these times.

There are four main types of crisis, namely (i) painful or infarctive, (ii) haemolytic, (iii) hypoplastic or aplastic and (iv) sequestration crises. Quite frequently, two or more types of crisis occur together in various combinations.

Infarctive crises

Painful crisis is the most common and results from infarction of the affected tissue, particularly bone. It most commonly affects the limbs (hands, feet and the digits in infancy and early childhood, and arms and legs in older children). It may last a few hours, days or sometimes weeks. The end of painful crisis may be as abrupt and unpredictable as the start. The pain may be extremely severe and stabbing or may be a prolonged dull ache. (A well educated patient, a mother of four children, said that pain in some attacks was more severe than that of childbirth.) It is important to appreciate the severity of pain in some of these attacks in order to relieve it effectively with appropriate analgesics.

Some of the infarctive crises are associated with non-pitting oedematous swelling of the limbs which may be complicated by abscesses in the soft tissues or by osteomyelitis. In a vast majority of crises, however, there are no sequelae after the attack.

Haemolytic crises

Haemolysis accompanies pain quite frequently. This may cause more intense jaundice, severe anaemia and congestive cardiac failure. In some instances, haemolytic crises occur without pain. In the usual haemolytic crisis, response by the bone marrow is shown by a high reticulocytosis (reticulocyte count 5 to 50 per cent).

Hypoplastic crises

In hypoplastic crisis, however, the anaemia is not accompanied by a reticulocytosis, and bone marrow biopsy may show actual inactivity. Hypoplastic crises, though quite uncommon in our experience, are usually precipitated by severe bacterial infection.

Sequestration crises
Severe anaemia is also a prominent feature of acute sequestration, but anaemia here is caused by trapping of the erythrocytes in large numbers in the spleen and the liver within a short time, resulting in sudden enlargement of these organs. Sequestration crises may result in death from congestive cardiac failure if red cells are not quickly and carefully transfused, as discussed under management. Sequestration crises are comparatively rare in childhood and more commonly reported in pregnancy (see Ch. 7).

Anaemia
Anaemia is a usual, but by no means an invariable, feature of sickle-cell disease. At the time of presentation of about 2000 Nigerian patients, 16 per cent of children with sickle-cell anaemia and five per cent of those with Hb-SC disease had haematocrit values (PCV) of 0·07 to 0·15 and therefore required emergency blood transfusion (Table 5.4). Thirty-eight per cent of Hb-SS and eight per cent of Hb-SC children presented with moderate anaemia (PCV < 0·20). However, 13 per cent of Hb-SS and 28 per cent of Hb-SC patients had a PCV of 0·31 or above.

Table 5.4   Haematocrit (PCV) distribution at the time of presentation of children with Hb-SS and Hb-SC disease.

PCV	Hb-SS % of total	Hb-SC % of total
0·07–0·15	16	5
0·16–0·20	22	3
0·21–0·25	24	16
0·26–0·30	25	48
0·31–0·35	9	17
0·36–0·40	4	11

Most of these children in the steady state have a PCV of 0·18 to 0·30 over a period of many years and are usually quite active. A dramatic drop of PCV during a crisis may, however, cause severe anaemia and congestive heart failure. Anaemia is haemolytic in type, but will be complicated by folate deficiency if supplements are not given. Low serum iron concentrations have been demonstrated in some Nigerian patients (Oluboyede, O.A., personal communication), but interpretation of this finding is not yet clear.

Bone marrow and bones

Abnormalities of bone marrow and bone arise from two mechanisms: (i) erythroid hyperplasia and (ii) infarction.

Erythroid hyperplasia leads to varying degrees of bossing of the bones of the skull (see Fig. 5.1) and to gnathopathy in almost all patients, except those with a very mild haemolytic process, which is more usual in Hb-SC disease (see Ch. 8).

In infancy and early childhood (six months to two years), most infarctive crises involve the hands and feet. In older children, the long bones are frequently involved.

Dactylitis and the hand-foot syndrome

The digits (particularly the fingers and less frequently the toes) become inflamed, that is hot, swollen, painful and tender (dactylitis). Involvement of the digits is commonly bilateral and symmetrical.

The soft tissues of the dorsa of the hands and feet are frequently involved bilaterally in this inflammatory process, causing the 'hand-foot syndrome'. Although both hands and feet are commonly affected at the same time, sometimes only the hands or the feet may be inflamed. Dactylitis and the hand-foot syndrome occur frequently together (Fig. 5.2), but each may occur independently of the other.

About 90 per cent of patients aged two years and below present with either dactylitis, hand-foot syndrome or a combination of

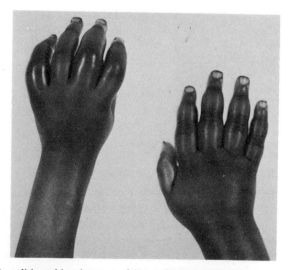

Fig. 5.2 Dactylitis and involvement of dorsa of both hands in a 9-month-old baby with Hb-SS.

both. While the non-pitting inflammatory swellings of the dorsa of hands and feet are almost pathognomonic of sickle-cell disease, dactylitis occurs in other, much less common conditions, such as Still's disease (juvenile rheumatoid arthritis), tuberculosis and congenital syphilis. It is easy to differentiate sickle-cell dactylitis from Still's disease, as the swellings in the former most commonly involve the proximal and middle phalanges (see Fig. 5.2) while in the latter the proximal interphalangeal joints are affected. Dactylitis in Still's disease is chronic and persistent while that of sickle-cell disease is usually a short-lived phenomenon. As dactylitis is rare in both tuberculosis and syphilis, it needs no further comments here.

Involvement of the hands and feet usually clears completely, but if infarction is severe it may be complicated by abscesses in the soft tissue, by osteomyelitis or by both. It is therefore advisable that investigations should include blood culture and X-ray of the affected limb to determine whether or not such infections exist. It should be noted, however, that it is difficult to differentiate infarction from osteomyelitis radiologically in the early stages. As in other types of crises, fever is a regular feature of hand-foot syndrome and dactylitis.

Long-term complications of dactylitis and the hand-foot syndrome are shortening and deformities of some fingers or toes.

Infarcts in other bones
Many older children complain of chronic aches and pains in the limbs, spine and head, with more severe episodes occurring at intervals which vary from about once a week to once a year. Infarcts in bone usually resolve completely in a few days or weeks. In a few patients, however, there is permanent damage, such as aseptic necrosis of the femoral neck (unilateral or bilateral), resulting in a waddling gait, or arrest of growth of the affected bone with consequent shortening of one of the lower limbs. Not many children show clinical features of aseptic necrosis, but radiologists make the diagnosis frequently, and it seems that this complication is often asymptomatic at this age.

Osteomyelitis
A more common complication of bones is osteomyelitis. Acute osteomyelitis in sickle-cell disease frequently presents as septicaemia, and the children are desperately ill, pyrexial, toxic and deeply jaundiced. Jaundice in such children has a high fraction of conjugated bilirubin, and clinically there are greenish-yellow sclera and dark urine containing bile. This jaundice can be confused easi-

ly with that of viral hepatitis. It is with close physical examination, that a hot and tender swelling or multiple swellings will be found on the limbs. There may also be associated pneumonia, and a blood culture at this stage will usually yield one of the Salmonella group of organisms. Multiple small abscesses may be found in children with septicaemia and sickle-cell disease.

The more common mode of presentation of osteomyelitis in these children, however, is in the follow-up clinic with chronic lesions, such as discharging sinuses. It is worthwhile to mention certain characteristics of osteomyelitis in sickle-cell disease.

1. In most patients it is multifocal, affecting the whole length of many bones, and is frequently symmetrical.

2. Unlike acute staphylococcal osteomyelitis, growing points of the bones or metaphysial plates are not the sites of predilection even at the initial stages.

3. In a large proportion of patients, the disease runs a chronic and prolonged course and the children do not appear as ill as one would expect, considering the number of bones affected.

4. Salmonella organisms are a frequent enough cause of osteomyelitis in sickle-cell disease to make the use of chloramphenicol a routine while culture results are being awaited.

Salmonella organisms are uncommon causes of osteomyelitis generally, but of 63 children with Salmonella osteomyelitis diagnosed in Ibadan, the haemoglobin electrophoretic patterns were 57 Hb-SS, one Hb-SC, one Hb-AS, two Hb-S/HPHF and only two Hb-AA (Adeyokunnu and Hendrickse, 1980). Half the patients were children under three years of age. The Salmonellae isolated included *S. typhi*, *S. paratyphi*, *S. typhimurium* and other species. In 32 of the 63 patients, other organisms were cultured from the blood or pus, the most common of which were *Staph. pyogenes* and coliforms.The lesions were bilaterial in the majority of patients, and the most common sites were hands and feet in children under age of two years and the long bones in older children.

In 30 patients with pathological fractures seen at Ibadan during one year (1974 to 1975), sickle-cell disease was found to be the most common single predisposing factor, accounting for nine (30 per cent) in those below 20 years of age (Ebong, 1978).

The laboratory investigation of suspected osteomyelitis in sickle-cell disease includes the culture of blood and pus (if any), haematological studies (including PCV, white cell and reticulocyte count), and X-ray of the chest and the limbs involved.

A combination of chloramphenicol (80 mg/kg/day) and cloxacillin or erythromycin have been found to be effective within four to six weeks in most patients. These antibiotic combinations may be changed if culture and sensitivity results so indicate. As many infections pursue a prolonged course and may lead to limb deformities (Fig. 5.3), the children should be managed with the help of orthopaedic surgeons. Surgical intervention, such as sequestrectomy, is however, rarely undertaken.

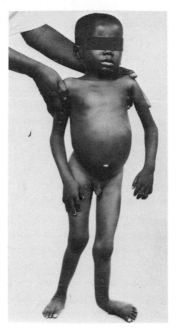

Fig. 5.3 Deformity of left leg following chronic osteomyelitis in a boy with sickle-cell anaemia.

The liver and spleen

Jaundice
Mild to moderate jaundice is common in sickle-cell disease. In contrast to the common haemolytic jaundice, the obstructive type is encountered less frequently. Patients with obstructive jaundice are usually above six years old, have an enlarged firm or hard liver and less frequently an enlarged spleen. Some of these children have clubbing of the digits of varying degrees of severity; there is no obvious explanation for this, but it is suggested that finger clubbing in sickle-cell disease is due to liver cell damage and cholestasis rather than respiratory causes. Abnormal liver function tests have been reported by many authors, including Hendrickse (1960), and in most of the patients with clubbing studied so far, cirrhosis of the

liver has been demonstrated histologically (unpublished observations).

Hepatosplenomegaly

Enlargement of the liver and spleen are common features and should be considered together, as they have essentially a common aetiology. Hepatosplenomegaly is due mainly to chronic haemolysis, but results occasionally from acute sequestration of red cells. About 70 per cent of Hb-SS children have splenic enlargement at the time of presentation; splenomegaly is much less frequent in Hb-SC children. Splenomegaly may vary widely in size from a few centimetres to gross enlargement in which the edge reaches the iliac fossa. The spleen is usually quite soft in consistency in early childhood, but becomes hard later. Tenderness over the splenic area (as a result of infarction) is quite common during abdominal crisis. There may be hypersplenism in some patients, with resultant more intractable anaemia, neutropoenia and thrombocytopoenia; splenectomy may prove beneficial in a few patients.

The liver is palpably enlarged in about 50 per cent of patients when first seen. This proportion increases appreciably as the children grow older, and the consistency changes from soft to firm or hard in some patients because of recurrent infarctions and haemosiderosis. The liver may be tender in a number of complications of sickle-cell disease, including (i) congestive cardiac failure from anaemia or cor pulmonale, (ii) infarctions during abdominal crisis and (iii) viral hepatitis, which is probably more common and more severe in these children.

Autosplenectomy

In both Hb-SS and Hb-SC, splenomegaly becomes less frequent with increasing age of the patients. This is due to siderofibrosis of the spleen which results from recurrent infarctions and iron deposition in this organ. The final result is a shrivelled fibrotic spleen (autosplenectomy). Autosplenectomy is reported to be almost universal in North American patients after the age of 10 years. However, massive spleens are found frequently in African children well above this age, and it is suggested that persistence of splenomegaly in these patients is due to endemic malaria.

Functional asplenia (defined as impaired splenic reticuloendothelial function in children with sickle-cell anaemia in spite of splenic enlargement) has been reported in young children; functional asplenia is associated with increased proneness to infection and may be reversed temporarily by the transfusion of fresh blood (Pearson et al., 1970).

Another infrequent splenic abnormality in sickle-cell disease is calcification, demonstrated by radiography usually in adults but only infrequently in children (see Ch. 8). There are no specific symptoms, and calcification is usually an accidental finding during radiographic investigation.

Involvement of other systems

Cardiovascular and respiratory systems

The heart is affected to a greater or lesser degree, depending on the severity of chronic anaemia and extent of recurrent pulmonary infarctions and infections. Cardiomegaly can be demonstrated in most patients after the age of about six years. All the chambers of the heart are usually involved, but the right ventricle and pulmonary artery will be more prominent when there is associated chronic pulmonary disease. Clinically, cardiomegaly can be demonstrated in many; haemic murmurs are common, and in a smaller number of patients there may be apical murmurs similar to those of chronic rheumatic heart disease. In patients with pulmonary hypertension, a parasternal heave and an accentuated pulmonary second heart sound are important physical signs. The heart fails quite frequently during crisis from severe anaemia or chest infection. This should always be borne in mind so as to insitute appropriate therapy.

The respiratory system is frequently affected by infection and infarctions. Pneumonia in sickle-cell disease is usually bronchopneumonia rather than lobar in type. It may persist longer than in children with normal haemoglobin despite intensive antibiotic therapy. This is most probably due to devitalisation of pulmonary tissue from infarction preceding the infections. In some cases, what appears radiologically to be pneumonic consolidation may actually be an infarct. Treatment should be with a broad spectrum antibiotic, such as ampicillin or chloramphenicol, over long periods. Although we have not found a higher frequency of pulmonary tuberculosis in these children, it is prudent to think of this when pneumonia fails to resolve after adequate therapy with antibiotics.

Infections in other systems

In our experience, bacterial infections in sickle-cell disease are less common at other sites than the respiratory and skeletal systems. Fulminant pneumococcal infections and meningitis have been reported in many studies from the United States of America (Barrett-

Connor, 1971); in one report, pneumococcal meningitis was 20 times as common in children with sickle-cell anaemia as in those with normal haemoglobin (Kabins and Lerners, 1970). In a review of pneumococcal meningitis in 114 Nigerian children aged 10 years and below (Nottidge, 1980), haemoglobin electrophoresis results were available for 54 patients; of these, 11 (20·4 per cent) were Hb-SS and one was Hb-SC. Since not more than 1 per cent of children surviving to this age are expected to have Hb-SS, the figure of 20 per cent agrees with the report from America (Kabins and Lerners, 1970). Pneumococcal meningitis and septicaemia occur predominantly in children under three years of age.

Malarial infection with *P. falciparum* is less intense in Hb-SS than in normal individuals, but the consequences of infection are severe. It is a frequent precipitating cause of crisis (haemolytic, sequestration and infarctive) and a common cause of death in both Hb-SS and Hb-SC disease.

Central nervous system
The central nervous system is frequently affected. Complications occur usually during crises following occlusion, infarction or haemorrhage into the meninges or the brain. This may result in convulsions, coma, monoplegia, hemiplegia or other paralyses. In some children, an initial attack may present clinically as repeated twitching of one arm which may leave it weak and paretic. The arm may recover partially or completely, or may be further weakened by repeated episodes. It may become completely paralysed, with contracture at the elbow. Sickle-cell disease is probably the most common cause of non-congenital hemiplegia in Nigerian children. Most of these children learn to live with their disability, but recurrent episodes may leave a few with multiple joint contractures, defective or complete loss of speech, and incontinence of urine and faeces. Disturbances of intellectual function occur but are uncommon among these patients. Cerebral episodes may sometimes be severe and extensive enough to cause prolonged coma which terminates fatally or leaves the patient bed-ridden.

Many therapeutic approaches have been tried in the management of cerebral episodes, but with poor results in the more severe cases. Treatment is difficult since one does not know in any particular patient whether the lesion is occlusive or haemorrhagic. This makes the use of heparin unwise. Repeated transfusions with Hb-AA blood have not been beneficial in the few Nigerian patients in which this has been tried. Physiotherapy must, however, be undertaken to prevent contractures and improve limb function. A simple but effective way in which to encourage a child to exercise a partly paralysed hand is to give the child a tennis ball to squeeze and play with.

Impairment or loss of sight and hearing are uncommon in children. In one two-year-old boy in our clinic, however, an acute febrile episode was complicated by deafness in both ears and this did not improve after a two-year follow up. Such children should be sent early to the school for the deaf.

Genitourinary system
The genitourinary system is almost invariably affected to some extent in patients with sickle-cell disease.

Frequently, the parents complain that their children have polyuria, nocturia and polydipsia. These tend to worsen with age as a result of the poor concentrating ability of the kidneys. It has been noted that intensive transfusion with Hb-AA blood is followed by temporary improvement of the concentrating function. Other defective functions, such as poor acidification of urine, have been reported.

Haematuria occurs in children with Hb-SS, Hb-SC and Hb-AS genotypes. Radiological studies on some 180 randomly selected Nigerian children with sickle-cell disease have shown calyceal abnormalities in a large proportion, necrotising papillitis in some and bilateral enlargement of the kidneys in a few (Daini, S.S.A., personal communication).

Priapism occurs in male children even under eight years of age, but the complication is rare at this age; its management is discussed in Chapter 6. Prognosis is unfortunately bad, and none of 15 Nigerian children with priapism reported any erection during the following two years (Adeyokunnu, A.A. and Lawani, J., personal communication). Other genital complications are delay in maturation of external genitalia in both male and female, delayed puberty and hypogonadism.

MANAGEMENT OF SICKLE-CELL DISEASE

Maintaining good health
The aim is to maintain the child in a reasonable state of good health, make his attendance at school as regular as possible and prolong his useful and enjoyable life. Some time should be spent during the first visit explaining the aetiology and natural history of the disease to the parents. In a less busy clinic, this can be done by a medical social worker or a nurse who has full understanding of

the disease and the mechanism of its inheritance. The parents are instructed to protect the child from inclement weather, to feed him well, to prevent excessive exertion, but not to treat him as an invalid. They should be told that they must not expect too much of the child in the line of physical or athletic achievement. They are instructed to bring the child to the hospital at any time of the day or night that he falls ill. At the first consultation, investigations should include PCV, reticulocyte count, blood film, total white cell and differential counts, urinalysis, haemoglobin electrophoresis, X-ray of the chest for assessment of the size of the heart, and X-ray of any affected bones, if seen during a crisis.

After the first two follow-up visits, the child should be seen once every two or three months in the case of sickle-cell anaemia or every four to six months in Hb-SC disease. Long-term follow up can be carried out by experienced nurses who refer only patients in severe crisis or those with other problems to physicians.

Patients should be prescribed a curative course of chloroquine at their first attendance. The usual oral dosage is 10 mg chloroquine base per kg body weight on the first day, divided into two doses, followed by 5 mg per kg body weight for two days, also divided into two doses. If the patient is unable to take drugs by month, it will be necessary to give the first two doses of chloroquine by intramuscular injection, after which oral treatment can be given. At the first and every subsequent visit, all patients should be given prophylactic antimalarials, such as pyrimethamine (in weekly dosage ranging from 6·25 mg for infants and young children to 25 mg for adolescents) or proguanil (25 mg daily up to the age for two years, 50 mg daily from two to five years and 100 mg daily for children over five years). Whenever a patient has failed to take prophylactic antimalarials for more than one week, treatment should be restarted with a course of chloroquine.

Folic acid (5 mg daily) is given routinely to all patients of all ages. Iron must not be prescribed unless iron deficiency has been proven.

Treatment of crises
Treatment of crises depends on the type and severity.

Infarctive crises
Since pain is the most common symptom, emphasis should be placed on its relief. Analgesics must be used liberally when the pain is severe. Aspirin is the most commonly used minor analgesic; soluble aspirin is preferable if it is available. It can be given in doses as

high as 130 mg per kg body weight per 24 hours at four-to six-hourly intervals. Paracetamol or novalgin may be more effective. Oral pethidine can be given in 25 to 50 mg tablets three times a day for three days when severe pain is persistent. Pethidine should be administered intramuscularly when pain is severe enough to prevent sleep. No drug addiction has been encountered following such use.

Hydration must be maintained, and the patient should be encouraged to take fluids orally unless he is vomiting. If there is vomiting or the child is very sick, intravenous fluids are indicated, and these may include M/6 sodium lactate or 8·4 per cent sodium bicarbonate solutions to counteract acidosis, and 5 or 10 per cent dextrose to provide nutrition, or Darrow's solution.

Careful clinical examination and laboratory investigation for the possibility of infection should be undertaken, and antibiotics are given only when there is proven or strongly suspected infection. Therapeutic doses of chloroquine are always given in the routine management of crises, and prophylactic antimalarials and folic acid supplements are continued.

Anaemic crises
Anaemia should only be treated with blood transfusion if the haematocrit is very low (Hb < 4·5 g/dl or PCV < 0·15), or if anaemia is severe enough to cause heart failure. Transfusions should be given with the greatest possible care to sickle-cell children to avoid the danger of circulatory overload. The blood should be carefully cross-matched and only small amounts of concentrated red cells are transfused, sufficient to tide the patient over the acute period. Only blood with haemoglobin electrophoretic type AA should be transfused. Since the children may need repeated transfusions, there is danger of serum hepatitis, increased iron load with resultant haemosiderosis and liver damage, and sensitisation to red cell and other antigens; therefore, the number of blood transfusions should be kept to a necessary minimum. Treatment of malaria or bacterial infection alone will often result in a rapid rise of PCV from values as low as 0·13 to 0·20 in about three days.

PROGNOSIS

Though there are no statistics on survival, quality of life and mortality of children with sickle-cell disease from any clinic in West Africa, we are seeing a higher proportion of older patients now than 10 to 15 years ago. Many more of our patients are attending primary and secondary schools and competing favourably with children with normal haemoglobin. The universities and other institutions of higher learning now have a number of adult patients and a fair number are found in virtually all the professions. As these patients grow older, the frequency of crisis decreases to about one in six months, or even one in two or four years. The severity of crises also diminishes. However, tragic deaths do occur frequently from infections both in children and adults.

Improvement in the prognosis and quality of life experienced by these patients during the last decade cannot be attributed only to improved medical facilities. The most important factor has been a rise in the socio-economic standard of living of the population. It is expected that with further improvement in living conditions, including higher standards of hygiene, life expectancy of these patients will increase considerably during the coming decade.

FURTHER READING

Adeyokunnu, A.A & Hendrickse, R.G. (1980) Salmonella osteomyelitis in childhood. A report of 63 cases seen in Nigerian children of whom 57 had sickle-cell anaemia. *Archives of Disease in Childhood*, 55, 175–184.

Anonymòus (1978) Sickle-cell anaemia in infancy. *Lancet*, i, 1439.

Barrett-Connor, E. (1971) Bacterial infection and sickle-cell anemia. An analysis of 250 infections in 166 patients and a review of the literature. *Medicine*, 50, 97–112.

Ebong, W.W. (1978) Pathological fractures of long bones in Nigerian children and adolescents. *Nigerian Journal of Paediatrics*, 5, 16–19.

Hendrickse, R.G. (1960) Sickle-cell anaemia in Nigerian children. *Central African Journal of Medicine*, 6, 45–57.

Kabins, S.A. & Lerner, C. (1970) Fulminant pneumococcemia and sickle-cell anemia. *Journal of American Medical Association*, 211, 467–471.

Nottidge, V.A. (1980) Pneumococcal meningitis in Nigerian children. *Nigerian Journal of Paediatrics (in press)*.

Pearson, H.A. Cornelius, E.A. Schwartz, A.D. Zelson, J.H. Wolfson, S.L. & Spencer, R.P. (1970) Tranfusion-reversible functional asplenia in young children with sickle-cell anemia. *New England Journal of Medicine*, 283, 334–337.

Powars, D.R. (1975) Natural history of sickle cell disease — the first ten years. *Seminars in Hematology*, 12, 267–285.

Sickle-cell disease during and after puberty

The majority of African infants with sickle-cell disease are born in villages where still the transmission of malaria is intense, other infectious diseases are frequent and nutrition is poor. Only a few live more than two years; for example, in Garki District, Kano State, Nigeria, 2 per cent of infants were Hb-SS, but the prevalence fell to 0·4 per cent in children aged one to four years and to only 0·05 per cent (one individual) over the age of nine years. Whenever a haematology laboratory and a sickle-cell clinic are first opened in an area of tropical Africa previously untouched by modern medicine, not many Hb-SS patients will be seen who have reached puberty; these few will be in poor health and show many of the chronic and acute complications of sickle-cell disease. However, the character of the 'adult' sickle-cell clinic will change rapidly in the first few years as it becomes common for the diagnosis to be made early in life, and children are given adequate treatment and then transferred to the adult clinic in good health.

SICKLE-CELL ANAEMIA (Hb-SS)

Growth and development
Children with Hb-SS are below average height, but bone maturation is usually normal up to 11 years. After that age, skeletal maturation is delayed and bone age is commonly less than actual age. Fusion of the epiphyses is late and may not be complete until after 20 years of age. This allows growth to continue for longer than normal so that Hb-SS subjects often eventually reach average height, or even go on to above average; young men are seen occasionally who are 190 cm (6 ft 3 in) or more in height.

Puberty is delayed. In girls, the menarche occurs on average one year later than in the normal population; menstruation is often irregular for up to the first 18 months. Young patients of both sexes should be reassured that they may expect full normal sexual development but that this is likely to be later than in their friends.

Adult habitus

The variation of body build is wide, from dwarfism to near-giantism. Typically, adults with sickle-cell anaemia are slender, with narrow shoulders and hips; the arms, hands, fingers, legs, feet and toes are long and thin. The neck often appears short and the normal curvatures of the spine are pronounced. The trunk is small for the total height, so that sitting height is below average while standing height is average or above average. The chest is deep (anteroposterior measurement) and narrow (lateral measurement), giving a hoop-chested appearance. Weight is low on average, and there is little body fat, possibly due to malabsorption.

Sickle-cell anaemia in the steady state

A patient with sickle-cell anaemia diagnosed for the first time after childhood is likely to have had a moderately severe history; a few patients present for the first time well into adult life, when the diagnosis is liable to overlooked. The commonest complaint is of severe aching pain in the bones; usual sites are the bones around the joints of the limbs; episodes recur typically about once a month and last five days to one week. Patients with the mildest disease may complain of 'occasional rheumatism' or only admit to infrequent pains after direct and insistent questioning. Pains are more frequent when the weather is wet or cold. The second commonest complaint is of abdominal pain. Other symptoms include headache, chest pain, epistaxis, episodes of jaundice, general weakness, breathlessness on exertion or any of the complications described below.

Scarification or tattooing is seen frequently over the heart, the spleen and various bones in patients who have been treated by traditional tribal medicine (Konotey-Ahulu, 1974).

Skeletal changes

Erythroid hyperplasia leads to expansion of the bone marrow cavity and bossing of the bones of the skull. Characteristically, the forehead is rounded with exaggeration of the supraorbital sulci, and there is expansion of the maxilla causing forward protrusion of the upper incisor teeth (gnathopathy) which can range from the teeth being slightly exposed at rest to their being almost horizontal. Bossing of the vault of the skull is not so common, but in extreme instances the head is grossly enlarged and the outer table so thin as to be easily depressed by gentle pressure, causing great pain. Gross bossing is largely reversible with protection against malaria and folic acid supplements; as it is not seen in non-malarial countries, it is probably the result of even greater erythroid hyperplasia induced by malarial haemolysis.

Skeletal changes resulting from both erythroid hyperplasia and infarction are discussed in detail in Chapter 8.

Anaemia and jaundice

The range of haemoglobin concentration shown by patients in the steady state is wide (Table 6.1); females have only a slightly lower average haemoglobin than males with Hb-SS. Certain patients live with a haemoglobin of less than 7·0 g/dl without any more disadvantage than those with a haemoglobin of 10 g/dl; the compensatory mechanisms of increased cardiac output and oxygen release through high intraerythrocyte 2,3-DPG allow the patients to remain without breathlessness at rest, but with greatly impaired reserves. Reticulocyte counts range from 2 to 20 per cent.

Table 6.1   Haemoglobin concentration (95 per cent confidence range) in Jamaican adults with sickle-cell disease in the steady state. (From Bannerman *et al.*, 1979; Serjeant *et al.*, 1979).

	Number	Hb g/dl Male	Number	Female
Hb-SS	60	6·0–9·6	63	5·9–9·9
Hb-SC	15	11·2–16·7	16	9·6–13·9
Hb-S/β°thal	20	6·6–10·7	21	6·7–10·3

Bilirubin production is about six times normal so that the serum bilirubin is 35 to 140 μmol/l (2 to 8 mg/dl) in the steady state. Cholelithiasis can be demonstrated in about one third of adult American patients, but in only about 10 per cent of Nigerian patients (Akinyanju and Ladapo, 1979). It is possible that the lower frequency in Nigerians is related to a diet rich in fibre. Symptoms from these pigment stones are not usual.

The reticuloendothelial system

Lymphadenopathy. Cervical lymph nodes are palpable in almost all children or adolescents seen for the first time; no specific cause is found in most patients. If there are other signs of active upper respiratory tract infection, the nodes usually diminish following a short course of antibacterial therapy, such as co-trimoxazole for five days. Inguinal lymph nodes are invariably palpable even in normal subjects who go barefoot.

The spleen. The balance between factors causing splenomegaly (congestion with sickled cells and malaria) and factors causing shrinkage of the spleen (sickle-cell infarct and acquired immunity to malaria) results in the spleen being palpable in only about 7 per cent of African patients by the age of puberty. Splenic infarct is less and splenomegaly persists longer in patients with high Hb-F and few irreversibly sickled cells in the blood. The spleen is usually not more than 8 cm below the costal margin in its longest axis and is characteristically hard; in the occasional patient there is gross splenomegaly.

Hepatomegaly
It is almost invariable for the liver to be palpable up to 6 cm below the costal margin in African patients. The surface is smooth and consistency is normal. Occasionally the enlargement may be gross, reaching below the umbilicus, and right ventricular failure should be suspected in these patients.

Cardiovascular system
The heart is enlarged, and the apex beat is displaced laterally and may be visible. Pulsation of the pulmonary artery in the second left intercostal space is commonly palpable. The pulse rate is normal at rest but rapid after minimal exertion, excitement or apprehension. Mid-systolic murmers are heard in almost all patients; third heart sounds are common, but the presence of other abnormal clinical signs suggests that there are complications or additional disease.

Pulmonary system
The total lung capacity, vital capacity and other measurements of lung volume are reduced. In the steady state, there are no particular physical signs.

Renal system
Disruption of the renal medulla by sickling leads to an inability to concentrate urine. Patients may complain of polyuria and polydipsia; enuresis is uncommon at this age, but nocturia is usual.

Central nervous system
It is unusual for there to be impairment of cerebral or neurological function. Academic achievement may be poor because of loss of schooling through illness or over-protectiveness by parents, but some patients have completed university degree courses. Patients are generally remarkably well adapted, doing their work or sports up to their capability and stopping without fuss when they are no longer able to compete.

Maintaining the steady state

The condition should be explained to the patients or to the nearest adult relatives in such detail as is within their comprehension, and in a language in which they are fluent. This is done at their first clinic attendance and reinforced at later visits; a pamphlet can be issued in a language in which the patients or relatives are literate (see Appendix III). A family history will give an opportunity to trace siblings with sickle-cell disease.

The triggers to crisis are explained, and the patients are advised to avoid undue exertion and cold, especially at night and during the cold and wet season. Swimming is one sport which is inadvisable. A large intake of alcohol carries the risk of dehydration, but moderate intake may be permitted to those who like it. Generally, patients know their own limitations and live up to them; they are to be encouraged in this and to lead as near to normal lives as possible.

They are advised to report whenever they are unwell, either to a weekly sickle-cell clinic or to a doctor at any other time. Identification cards stating the diagnosis are of great value, allowing appropriate treatment to be started without delay and avoiding the repetition of laboratory investigations. Women are told to report as soon as they think they may be pregnant.

At first attendance, a curative dose of an antimalarial is prescribed; chloroquine 600 mg base as a single dose is adequate in the immune subject in Africa, where chloroquine resistance is still rare. Antimalarial prophylaxis is maintained; proguanil (Paludrine) 100 mg per day is a most satisfactory regime, as it is highly effective in Africa, is easily remembered and has few undesirable actions. Folic acid supplements 5 mg per day are given. Patients are supplied with aspirin (preferably soluble aspirin) and instructed to take up to four 300 mg tablets (according to body size) not more than four-hourly when they have pain of a severity not demanding hospital admission; it should be emphasised that aspirin is not a tonic to be taken indiscriminately, and patients are warned to stop treatment if they experience tinnitus. The simple regime of one proguanil and one folic acid tablet per day should not be burdened with other ineffective therapies; yeast and vitamin mixtures, for example, only add confusion and may deter patients from taking the two vital tablets. Iron deficiency is rare in sickle-cell patients in Africa, and iron should not be prescribed unless deficiency is proven. Patients should be warned against buying for themselves, often at great cost, useless 'tonics' (usually containing iron) or other medicaments.

Patients are asked to return to the clinic at 13-week intervals; the importance of regular attendance even when they remain in good health must be emphasised. On return visits, the number of painful crises or other episodes is recorded. Women are asked the date of their last menstrual period and examined to see whether they are pregnant if there has been amenorrhoea; any woman who is pregnant is referred to the obstetrician without delay (see Ch. 7). The patients are examined, but the collection of blood samples can be kept to a minimum and the haemoglobin estimation need not be repeated unless there is a suspicion of anaemic crisis.

If possible, social workers should be employed to find patients who have not kept their appointments, to discuss social problems and to give assistance when required. If a patient fails to take prophylactic antimalarials for more than one week, treatment should be started again with a curative dose of chloroquine.

Chronic complications of the steady state

The skeletal system

Avascular necrosis. The hand-foot syndrome in early childhood can cause premature epiphyseal fusion with shortening and distortion of the metacarpal and metatarsal bones in particular: there is irregular shortening of the toes and the fingers, with uneven knuckles when the fist is clenched.

Avascular necrosis of head of the femur causes severe disruption of the hip joint. Compression fractures of vertebral bodies are also crippling, but fortunately these complications are rare in Africa. Avascular necrosis of the head of the humerus, or of other bones which are not weightbearing, does not result in severe symptoms requiring orthopaedic treatment.

Osteomyelitis. Bone destruction by infarction is complicated by infection in less than 10 per cent of patients. Osteomyelitis arises acutely before five years of age in nearly half of the patients, and is seen as a chronic problem in the postpaediatric age, the long bones of the arms and legs being the most common sites affected. Treatment, which is by surgical drainage and chloramphenicol, ampicillin or other antibiotics according to organisms isolated, is unrewarding and recurrence is usual.

Cardiopulmonary complications

Recurrent pulmonary infarction leads to interstitial fibrosis, pulmonary vascular obliteration and pulmonary hypertension; this can progress to enlargement of the right ventricle and chronic cor pulmonale. Patients are usually over 20 years of age; they are seriously incapacitated by dyspnoea, and examination shows a raised jugular venous pressure, pronounced enlargement of the liver, a loud second pulmonary heart sound over the second left intercostal space and enlargement of the right side of the heart. There may be finger clubbing. Oedema is not seen commonly in right-sided heart failure, possibly because of the diuretic action of sickle-cell disease itself. Digitalis is not often effective and diuretics are contraindicated unless there is salt and water retention. Treatment is supportive, including such measures as the treatment of pulmonary infections.

Gross splenomegaly

Gross splenomegaly persists in a small number of patients into adult life. The presence of Howell-Jolly bodies and nucleated red cells in the peripheral blood shows that these spleens are usually hypofunctional. Treatment with antimalarials results in a slight decrease in size only. If there are no symptoms or evidence of hypersplenism, no other treatment is indicated; splenectomy is hazardous and useless.

If there is severe anaemia and low neutrophil and platelet counts, red cell survival studies using radioactive chromium should be performed. Only if excessive red cell sequestration and haemolysis are demonstrated in the spleen, should splenectomy be considered in these rare patients.

Central nervous system

Acute infarctions, haemorrhage, emboli and meningitis are seen during childhood and only infrequently after 14 years. The late sequelae include hemiplegia, loss of cerebral function and a variety of neurological disorders.

Although most patients with unimpaired intelligence are remarkably self-reliant, a few become emotionally dependent on particular doctors, or on institutions such as the hospital or some unusual religious community.

Dwarfism

A limited number of patients have extreme retardation of growth and maturity, possibly related to the severity of sickle-cell disease itself, frequent recurrent infections (especially malaria) and malnutrition (folate deficiency may have an important role). Patients over the age of 20 years present with a clinical appearance similar to that of pituitary dwarfism, and the females complain of primary amenorrhoea. There is often a dramatic response to the administration of prophylactic antimalarials and folic acid supplements. There is a spurt of growth for about six months, but then the epiphyses fuse. Sexual maturation continues and becomes normal in both sexes.

Acute complications

Bone pain crisis

Onset is rapid, with severe, aching pain which is described as being in the bones. The patient may be weeping, moaning or screaming, and assuming grotesque postures. The common sites are the long bones of the limbs, the lumbar spine (loin or abdominal pain), the thoracic cage (chest pain) and the bones of the face. The hands and feet are not often affected after childhood.

There is usually little to be detected except fever, and warmth and tenderness over the affected bone. If there is swelling, redness and heat (rather than warmth), acute osteomyelitis is to be suspected, but this is unusual at this age. The bones of the face are exceptional, as there is considerable soft tissue swelling without infection of the underlying bone. Blood cultures should be performed in an attempt to confirm acute osteomyelitis and to identify the causative organism; radiographic appearances do not distinguish between acute infarction and osteomyelitis.

Search should be made for any infections which may be triggering the crisis. These include malaria and infections of the respiratory, gastrointestinal and urinary tract. The haemoglobin is unaltered during bone pain crisis, raised by dehydration or lowered by infection; the neutrophil and platelet counts are high.

Treatment. Patients with severe pain should be admitted to hospital. There is as yet no specific treatment proven to shorten the duration of crisis. A curative dose of chloroquine is given on the assumption that the patient has not been taking prophylactic antimalarials; proguanil and folic acid supplements are continued. Analgesics should be administered liberally, for example pethidine up to 100 mg intramuscularly (depending on body weight) every four hours. Too much emphasis has been laid on the risk of addiction, yet no Nigerian patient with sickle-cell anaemia has become dependent on opiates in a personal experience of about 15 years. Strong analgesics are decreased and withdrawn as soon as is humane, and the milder analgesics (for example aspirin) substituted.

Patients are often dehydrated and are therefore encouraged to drink, but it is often necessary to restore and maintain fluid balance with intravenous fluids. These should include M/6 sodium lactate in order to counteract metabolic acidosis, and dextrose 5 to 10 per cent as a source of nutrition.

Antibiotics are not indicated in most episodes of crisis, and their prescription should be kept to a minimum. Definite indications include (i) overt infections, such as urinary tract infection, (ii) suspected or proven acute osteomyelitis, which must be treated vigorously with, for example, chloramphenicol or ampicillin for up to three weeks, and (iii) high fever persisting for more than thirty-six hours. In the latter case, it is usual to prescribe a broad spectrum antibiotic, such as co-trimoxazole, but there have been no properly conducted trials, and it is doubtful whether patients do benefit in fact.

Severe infarction may be complicated by bone marrow necrosis and fat embolus to the lungs and cerebrum; diagnosis is made in life by staining the sputum with Sudan red and observing fat globules. The complication is more common in pregnancy. Good results are claimed for treatment by heparin (see Ch. 7), but no controlled trial has been performed.

Acute chest pain

Episodes of acute pain in the chest may arise from:

1. pulmonary infarction
2. pneumonia
3. infarction in the bones of the thoracic cage
4. angina (extremely rarely).

Physical examination will reveal if the source of pain is confined to the bones and that the lungs are apparently unaffected. Patients with sickle-cell anaemia are liable to acute pulmonary infarction and are very susceptible to pneumococcal and other types of pneumonia. The symptoms, signs and radiological appearances are almost indistinguishable in the two conditions. In some patients (mostly children) a causative organism is isolated and there is the rapid recovery with antibiotics typical of acute pneumonia, but in the majority of patients these acute pulmonary episodes are a combination of infection and infarction, and it is immaterial which came first. In spite of adequate broad spectrum antibiotic therapy, cough and fever may persist and resolution be delayed, usually for about one week.

Acute abdominal pain

Causes of acute pain in the abdomen include:

1. infarction in the mesentery
2. splenic infarction
3. infarction in the lumbar spine
4. duodenal ulcer and its complications
5. acute cholecystitis
6. obstruction of the cystic or bile ducts
7. pancreatitis
8. abdominal crises unrelated to sickle-cell disease.

There are no localising signs in the majority of patients, but careful abdominal palpation is essential to exclude splenic infarction (tenderness in the left hypochondrium over a palpable spleen), gallbladder pathology (tenderness over the right hypochondrium) or appendicitis (tenderness in the right iliac fossa). Tenderness localised in the hypogastrium or centrally suggests duodenal ulceration or pancreatitis, both of which can result from sickle-cell infarction; serum amylase estimation and barium meal radiography are then indicated.

The majority of crises of abdominal pain resolve in about five days on treatment with analgesics and maintenance of fluid intake. Splenic infarcts are rare at this age and no specific treatment is required (see also air travel below). Acute cholecystitis and obstruction of either the cystic duct or the common bile duct are infrequent, although pigment stones may be present in some patients (see above). Cholecystectomy is rarely necessary.

Duodenal ulceration. The incidence of duodenal ulceration increases with age and has been reported to be as high as 30 per cent in males over 25 years in Jamaica (Serjeant, 1974); women do not seem to suffer often from this complication. No series has been studied in Africa, but it is a common problem in adult males. The ulceration is certainly due to sickle-cell infarction, and the patients have normal gastric acidity.

As long as the course is uncomplicated, medical treatment is the same as that for duodenal ulcers in non-sickle-cell patients. The commonest acute presentation in the Nigerian experience is pyloric stenosis for which gastro-enterostomy will be required. Haematemesis is an infrequent complication.

Complications in the genitourinary system

Haematuria. Infarction causes ulceration of the renal pelvis which may progress to papillary necrosis. Bacteriuria and haematuria are not infrequent complications. Haematuria is characteristically painless, but the passage of clots may cause renal colic, which is usually unilateral. The left kidney is affected four times as commonly as the right. Renal biopsy should not be attempted. Patients are treated with intravenous M/6 sodium lactate to increase the urinary output; bacteriuria is treated with appropriate antibiotics. Aspirin should be avoided because it inhibits platelet function; the antifibrinolytic agent epsilon aminocaproic acid (EACA) is inadvisable in sickle-cell disease, but has been used successfully in haematuria in sickle-cell trait. Blood transfusion is indicated if there is shock or life-threatening anaemia.

Nephrectomy is the last resort when persistent haemorrhage is endangering the patient's life.

Priapism. Priapism is a persistent and painful penile erection with engorgement of the corpora cavernosa but not the corpus spongiosum, so that the glans penis remains flaccid. It is seen most commonly in adolescent and young adult males with sickle-cell disease and is brought on by sexual excitement or, rarely, by dysuria, but may occur spontaneously.

Mild priapism may last up to four hours and be relieved by micturition, walking around and bathing in cold water.

Moderately severe priapism will usually respond within 24 hours to bed rest, sedation, analgesics and hydration with intravenous M/6 sodium lactate.

In severe attacks, the penis is hot and exquisitely tender; pain is referred to the perineum and lower abdomen. If untreated, there is a gradual subsidence over about two weeks, with fibrosis of the corpora cavernosa and consequent impotence. Initial therapy should include pethidine or morphine and rehydration. Under general or spinal anaesthetic, a wide-bore needle (14 to 16 gauge) is inserted into the lateral surface of the base of the penis, and the dark viscous blood aspirated; this is followed by repeated irrigation with either saline or 10 per cent heparin and by aspiration until only fresh blood is obtained. The opinion of a urosurgeon should be sought, but surgery is not often recommended.

Leg ulceration

One of the most common complications of sickle-cell anaemia in the West Indies and America is leg ulceration. The ulcers start most often between 10 and 20 years of age, and the cumulative frequency in Jamaican adults is 76 per cent (Serjeant, 1974). Remarkably, not more than 5·4 per cent of West African patients over 12 years of age develop ulcers. Reasons for this relative immunity are not clear, but a higher intake of zinc in the food has been suggested (Akinyanju and Akinsete, 1979). African males are affected six times as often as females.

The ulcers are usually on the lower third of the leg, above the ankle and on the medial side; the left leg is affected more often than the right. The ulcers start as infarcts in the skin, causing small blister-like lesions; these develop into necrotic sloughs in about two weeks and then into ulcers less than 1 cm in diameter by about three weeks. Small ulcers may either heal or progress into ulcers up to 10 cm in diameter, with punched-out edges and a base of either red granulation tissue or yellow slough. Untreated, ulcers may heal slowly and irregularly with frequent breakdowns from trauma or infection, or an ulcer may spread further, involving bones and joints. Patients are liable to tetanus, especially if living in poor hygienic conditions. All patients are seriously incapacitated at work or at school.

Small, clean ulcers are relatively easily treated with daily antiseptic washing (Eusol) and dressing. Larger ulcers require in addition:

1. prolonged bed rest with the affected leg raised
2. bacteriological culture of the pus, followed by appropriate antibiotic therapy
3. hydrogen peroxide lotion or surgical debridement to remove the slough
4. blood transfusion to maintain the haemoglobin above 7·0 g/dl
5. tetanus prophylaxis.

A few patients with the largest ulcers, or those whose ulcers fail to heal, will require skin pinch grafts. It has been claimed that oral zinc sulphate 200 mg three times a day hastens healing. Once healed, the legs should be protected by wearing crêpe or elastic stockings.

Ocular lesions

In the steady state, retinal veins are tortuous and the arterioles show narrowing and later occlusion. This leads progressively to new vessel formation and *retinitis proliferans*. Adult patients, especially those with Hb-SC disease, may suffer transient monocular blindness or visual field defects from retinal haemorrhage, retinal detachment or vitreous haemorrhage. Vitreous haemorrhage needs no treatment, and the patient should be reassured that sight will recover over a period of up to six weeks. Retinal lesions should be referred to an ophthalmologist for treatment which may include laser beam coagulation.

Anaemic crisis

Departures from the steady-state haemoglobin levels are infrequent after childhood and are invariably the result of acute infections. Mechanisms of a rapidly falling haemoglobin include:

1. erythroid hypoplasia (aplastic crisis)
2. acute megaloblastic arrest of erythropoiesis
3. haemolytic crisis
4. sequestration crisis
5. malaria.

The course of viral or bacterial infection will be complicated by depression of the usually hyperactive bone marrow and by a rapid fall in the haemoglobin concentration and reticulocyte count. Depending on the nature of the infection, recovery of marrow function may be expected in five to ten days.

Pyrexia inhibits the activity of the enzyme dihydrofolate reductase, blocks normal folate metabolism and precipitates acute megaloblastic arrest of erythropoiesis in those patients who are not taking folic acid supplements and whose folate status is marginal. The haemoglobin concentration falls rapidly and profoundly.

An increase of the rate of haemolysis will result from most infections, but this is not more than contributory to the rapid decline of haemoglobin unless there is another factor, such as glucose-6-phosphate dehydrogenase deficiency or disseminated intravascular coagulation. Patients who have lost immunity to malaria by taking prophylactics and then stopping treatment are liable to acute *P. falciparum* infection and haemolysis. However, severe jaundice in an adult patient with sickle-cell disease is more likely to be the result of hepatitis than haemolysis.

Infection may be followed rarely by massive sequestration of red cells and rapid enlargement of the spleen in those adult patients who retain functional spleens; this is one complication where prompt transfusion of blood may be life-saving.

Anaemic crisis is managed by treatment of the precipitating infection, a curative dose of chloroquine followed by proguanil and folic acid supplements. There is usually a rapid return to the steady-state haemoglobin concentration without having to resort to blood transfusion.

Blood transfusion. Frequently patients with sickle-cell disease are given blood transfusions which are totally unnecessary. Transfusion should be kept to a minimum to avoid the risks of (i) hepatitis and other infections, (ii) sensitisation to cell and plasma antigens, making subsequent transfusions more difficult, and (iii) circulatory overload. Blood transfusion is indicated if the patient is in danger of anaemic cardiac failure, that is, if the haemoglobin is less than 4·0 g/dl, or less than 6·0 g/dl and falling rapidly. Blood is selected for cross-matching only after it has been shown to be Hb-AA by electrophoresis or at least to be not containing Hb-S by the solubility test. Preferably, it should have been stored for less than 48 hours since donation. Concentrated red cells, not whole blood, are transfused slowly with simultaneous intramuscular or intravenous injection of the rapidly acting diuretic frusemide, 40 mg for a 50 kg adult. In the severest anaemias (Hb < 3·0 g/dl), exchange blood transfusion is indicated (see Ch. 7).

Indications for blood transfusion other than for severe anaemia include haemorrhage, preparation for surgery, preparation for air travel and chronic leg ulceration.

Surgery
Emergency or elective surgery will be required both for conditions arising from sickle-cell anaemia (osteomyelitis, aseptic necrosis of bone, duodenal ulcers, cholelithiasis, leg ulceration, priapism) and for coincidental disease.

Patients may be prepared for major surgery by blood transfusion, giving Hb-AA concentrated cells from fresh blood with a rapidly acting diuretic. According to the initial haemoglobin concentration and the anticipated extent of surgery, a single transfusion of concentrated red cells from two units may be given, or this can be repeated at two- to three-day intervals until about half the circulating haemoglobin is Hb-A. An exchange blood transfusion may be necessary when major emergency surgery cannot be delayed.

Tourniquets should be avoided, as stasis leads to deoxygenation and sickling.

Whenever possible, local anaesthesia or nerve blocks should be employed. It is recommended that a general anaesthetic be preceded by five minutes oxygenation with 100 per cent oxygen and that there is hyperventilation with 30 to 50 per cent oxygen during anaesthesia (Homi *et al.*, 1979). Oxygen should be administered again in the postoperative phase until the patient has recovered full consciousness. The patient must be watched carefully during the first 36 hours after operation, as this is a time of danger of crisis. Hydration is maintained and acidosis prevented with intravenous M/6 sodium lactate; the haemoglobin concentration is raised above

7·0 g/dl by transfusion if necessary; oxygen is kept available at the bedside. The patient is mobilised as soon as possible.

Air travel

Commercial aircraft are pressurised to an atmosphere equivalent to about 2100 m (7000 ft), and the hypoxia experienced in both pressurised and unpressurised aircraft is sufficient to cause splenic infarction in some patients with sickle-cell disease, but not in normal subjects with sickle-cell trait.

The risk of splenic infarct seems to be greater in Hb-SC, Hb-S/ β-thal and other forms of sickle-cell disease than in Hb-SS, perhaps because the latter tend not to have functional spleens. The extent of the risk is not known; one boy with Hb-SS who flew from Nigeria to Australia via England, stopping only to change flights, experienced no discomfort and insisted on going to school the day after landing at Sydney.

Patients should be encouraged to travel by surface transport in preference to air flight when this is feasible. Against this advice must be weighed the risk of precipitating a crisis through fatigue, exposure to cold and dehydration, all of which are hazards of long journeys in uncertain vehicles on poor roads. Patients should undertake air travel only when they are in a steady state of health. It is usual to administer a transfusion of concentrated Hb-AA cells about five days before the flight, but whether this is beneficial or not is not clear. Patients should know how to call for oxygen if they have pain during the flight.

SICKLE–CELL-HAEMOGLOBIN C DISEASE

The pathology and clinical expression of Hb-SC disease are the same as those of Hb-SS but milder. Patients usually survive childhood, especially where the environmental factors improving prognosis prevail (see Table 4.1). Life expectancy is shortened certainly in females, because of the complications of pregnancy (see Ch. 7), and possibly in males, but the diagnosis has been made at over 80 years of age.

Patients may give a history of almost any of the complications discussed under Hb-SS, but to a milder extent. Adults with Hb-SC disease are usually of normal appearance, but the spleen is palpable in over 50 per cent of patients. There is haemolysis, and the haemoglobin concentration may be moderately low or normal (Table 6.1). The reticulocyte count is 1 to 7 per cent while the patient is in the steady state.

Two exceptions to the rule of a milder expression of Hb-SC than Hb-SS are that ocular complications are more apparent (possibly because of the higher haemoglobin concentration and the low solubility of Hb-C), and there seems to be a greater risk of splenic infarction during air travel.

Management
Hb-SC disease may be classified as severe, moderate or mild.

Patients with severe Hb-SC disease should be managed in the same manner as patients with Hb-SS. It should be remembered that the diagnosis may be incorrect in some patients said to have Hb-SC with severe expression. If the clinical picture is like that of Hb-SS and the blood film shows definite sickled cells, but the electrophoretic pattern suggests Hb-SC, the correct diagnosis may be Hb-SS + Hb-G-Philadelphia; the Hb-S solubility test gives an Hb-SS result in the latter condition (see Ch. 3).

Patients with moderately severe disease may be maintained on folic acid supplements alone. It is unlikely that these patients will attend the clinic regularly, and intermittent administration of prophylactic antimalarials will diminish acquired immunity to malaria. Every attempt must be made to persuade women in the reproductive period of life to keep attending the clinic so that pregnancy may be diagnosed early, antimalarials started and the patient referred to the obstetrician.

Males with mild disease probably need no treatment except when suffering from crises, which are usually minor and infrequent. The condition is explained to them and they are given identity cards. Females in the reproductive period of life should be urged to attend the clinic regularly and encouraged to do so by the administration of folic acid supplements, which are largely a placebo while they are not pregnant.

SICKLE-CELL-β-THALASSAEMIA

Sickle-cell-β°thalassaemia
Persons who inherit the genotype Hb-S/β°thal are likely to be misdiagnosed as having Hb-SS with high Hb-F (see Ch. 3). The symptoms, signs, growth development and anaemia (see Table 6.1) in Hb-S/β°thal are similar to those seen in Hb-SS, except that palpable splenomegaly persists in about 40 per cent of patients. Hypersplenism is common, and splenectomy may be indicated in about half of the patients with clinical splenomegaly (Serjeant et al., 1979).

Sickle-cell-β^+ thalassaemia

Persons who inherit the genotype Hb-S/β^+thal have symptoms of mild sickle-cell disease, but their haemoglobin electrophoretic pattern is liable to be mistaken for Hb-AS (see Ch. 3). The clinical expression and anaemia are mild. Management, as with Hb-SC, depends on the severity and frequency of symptoms.

REFERENCES

Akinyanju, O. & Akinsete, I. (1979) Leg ulceration in sickle-cell disease in Nigeria. *Tropical and Geographical Medicine*, **31**, 87–91.

Akinyanju, O. & Ladapo, F. (1979) Cholelithiasis and biliary tract disease in sickle-cell disease in Nigerians. *Postgraduate Medical Journal*, **55**, 400–402.

Bannerman, R.M., Serjeant, B., Seakins, M., England, J.M. & Serjeant, G.R. (1979) Determinants of haemoglobin level in sickle cell-haemoglobin C disease. *British Journal of Haematology*, **43**, 49–56.

Homi, J., Reynolds, J., Skinner, A., Hanna, W. & Serjeant, G. (1979) General anaesthesia in sickle-cell disease. *British Medical Journal*, i, 1599–1601.

Konotey-Ahulu, F.I.D. (1974) The sickle-cell diseases. *Archives of Internal Medicine*, **133**, 611–619.

Serjeant, G.R. (1974) *The Clinical Features of Sickle-Cell Disease*. Amsterdam: North-Holland.

Serjeant, G.R., Sommereux, AM., Stevenson, M., Mason, K. & Serjeant, B.E. (1979) Comparison of sickle-cell β° thalassaemia with homozygous sickle cell disease. *British Journal of Haematology*, **41**, 83–93.

Sickle-cell disease in pregnancy

Until recently, pregnancy in women with sickle-cell disease was comparatively rare because most of those affected died in infancy and childhood and many among the survivors remained subfertile. However, with steady improvements both in living standards and in health care, the picture is changing, and an increasing number of women with these diseases are reaching adulthood and their fertility continues to improve. Nevertheless, most of the problems they present during pregnancy, labour and the puerperium have remained the same. Severe anaemia, acute sequestration crises, bacterial infections, painful crises and pseudotoxaemia are the main complications, and they are partly responsible for the high maternal and fetal mortality associated with these diseases.

Maternal complications

Anaemia

There is often a great increase in the incidence and severity of anaemia during pregnancy, particularly in tropical Africa. This is not due to any intrinsic change in the haemolytic process, since red cell survival rates are the same in pregnant and non-pregnant subjects with sickle-cell disease. The increase in the severity of anaemia is often associated with three conditions: (i) folate deficiency, (ii) acute sequestration crises and (iii) malaria.

During pregnancy, folate deficiency leading to megaloblastic changes in the bone marrow is widely recognised wherever dietary intake is low and supplements are not given. Once the marrow becomes megaloblastic, the danger is that the anaemia may rapidly worsen and be fatal before appropriate treatment has time to take effect.

In acute sequestration crises, circulating red cells are trapped in the liver and spleen. One or both of these organs become enormous and the circulating haemoglobin level drops so precipitously that death from hypovolaemic shock may follow. For example, a fall in haemoglobin level from 10 g/dl to 6 g/dl within a few hours is common in these episodes. Acute sequestration crises may be precipitated by hypoxia, acidosis, venous congestion or infections, and they can occur at any period during pregnancy or labour, and in the puerperium, although the effects are most dangerous during labour.

In areas where *P. falciparum* is prevalent, the risk from anaemia is usually great. This is largely due to the fact that, in pregnancy, the maternal defences against malarial parasitaemia are lowered. Red cell destruction proceeds at an increased pace, and so must haemopoiesis if the haemoglobin concentration is to be maintained at a reasonable level. In the end, both the increased haemopoiesis and pregnancy itself further increase the demand for folic acid, and profound anaemia develops as a result of both haemolysis and megaloblastic erythropoiesis.

Painful crises

Painful crises are known to be precipitated by bacterial infections, fever, dehydration and acidosis. The pains occur at any time during pregnancy and labour, and in the puerperium. Any organ can be affected, but bones and joints are most commonly involved.

An important feature of painful crises in pregnancy is *pseudotoxaemia*, which refers to the appearance of systolic hypertension and proteinuria. It is associated with bone marrow fat embolism in the pulmonary vessels, and in the absence of effective treatment, mortality is very high indeed.

The last four weeks of pregnancy, together with all the stages of labour and the first four days of the puerperium, constitute the most dangerous period. Not only is the frequency of painful crises at this time higher than at any other period during pregnancy, but the pains are more severe, they last longer and they are more likely to be accompanied by pseudotoxaemia. Why this is, remains a mystery.

Infections

The important points to remember about infections in pregnant women with sickle-cell disease are that they are common, that they are much more difficult to control (especially in the puerperium) and that they are most severe when profound anaemia is present (Hb < 7 g/dl or PCV < 0·20). Furthermore, the fever and acidosis commonly associated with infection often worsen sickling and may thereby precipitate painful crises and acute sequestration.

Urinary and respiratory tract infections are the most frequent, but others, including salmonellosis, have also been found.

In the puerperium, wounds, both of the perineum and of the abdomen, frequently become septic. Poor maternal nutrition, severe anaemia, wound haematoma and local bacterial infections account for this, but another contributory factor is tissue hypoxia caused by sickling within the local capillaries. One danger of wound sepsis is that complete dehiscence may follow; in this case, satisfactory healing may require a prolonged period of hospitalisation even after secondary repair. The other danger of wound sepsis is that bacterial spread to other areas may be very rapid indeed. For example, septicaemia and intraperitoneal abscesses have been known to follow episiotomies and subcutaneous injection abscesses within a matter of days.

Pelvic deformities

Some women with sickle-cell disease may have an abnormal gait due to avascular necrosis of the femoral head and hip arthrodesis. Other abnormalities include android pelvis, straight sacrum and a general contraction of the pelvis, particularly in Hb-SS. These changes in the bony pelvis are thought to be the result of the poor somatic development of the mothers through the combined effects of chronic anaemia, frequent infections and poor nutrition. It is important to recognise these pelvic abnormalities early because of their adverse effects on the course and outcome of labour.

Maternal mortality

There is no doubt that in tropical Africa, where living standards are at present generally low, maternal mortality in sickle-cell disease is at least five times as high as in women with normal haemoglobin type. However, in parts of the United States of America and in the West Indies, with good nutrition and environmental hygiene, the outlook is better; maternal mortality in West Africa with the best available care is about 12 per cent in Hb-SS and 6 per cent in Hb-SC (Table 7.1).

The causes of maternal mortality in sickle-cell disease can be divided into two groups. The first consists of the complications associated with the disease itself, namely severe anaemia, bacterial infections, painful crises, pseudotoxaemia and acute sequestration. The second results from the fact that at the end of pregnancy, operative deliveries (which are more dangerous than easy spontaneous deliveries) are needed more often in patients with sickle-cell disease than in all others.

Although Hb-SS, Hb-SC and other sickle-cell diseases have similar clinical features, their prognoses in pregnancy differ: Hb-SS is

Table 7.1 Comparison of the frequency of complications in patients with normal haemoglobin type and others with sickle-cell disease attending antenatal clinic and delivering at University College Hospital, Ibadan, Nigeria (Harrison, 1976)

| | Haemoglobin types | | | |
	AA	SS	SC	S/β^+thal
Number of pregnancies	319	25	147	13
	% incidence within each group			
Anaemia (PCV < 0·30) (Hb < 10 g/dl)	20	92	45	60
Acute sequestration	0	24	2	0
Bone pain crises	0	70	50	8
Pseudotoxaemia	0	8	6	0
Pulmonary embolism	0	4	2	0
Preeclampsia during pregnancy	5	5	5	0
Preeclampsia in labour	5	22	7	0
Operative deliveries	10	52	10	8
Postpartum haemorrhage	2	2	3	23
Blood transfusion	14	44	16	8
Bacterial infections	11	52	30	15
Wound sepsis	6	55	10	0
Maternal deaths	0	12	6	0
No complications	42	0	33	8
Perinatal deaths/1000 deliveries	33	120	34	0

the most dangerous and Hb-S/β^+thal is the least hazardous (see Table 7.1).

Fetal prognosis

A high abortion rate and an increased perinatal mortality is characteristic of sickle-cell disease, especially in Hb-SS, where half of all viable pregnancies may end as stillbirths and early neonatal deaths. Most fetal deaths are the result of low birthweight, birth trauma and intrapartum asphyxia. With improvements in maternal and fetal care, perinatal deaths (see Table 7.1) have been reduced to 12 to 28 per cent in Hb-SS, 7 per cent in Hb-S/β °thal and 4 per cent in Hb-SC (Serjeant et al., 1979). Fetal complications are few when the mother has Hb-S/β^+thal (see Table 7.1).

Danger to the fetus is increased if there is any degree of intrapartum asphyxia, such as occurs in prolonged labour, with maternal anaemia, in preeclampsia and hypertension, and in antepartum haemorrhage. Even in the absence of these obstetric complications, the danger of asphyxia with sudden fetal death still persists.

Lastly, mothers with Hb-SS, but not those with other forms of sickle-cell disease, produce babies who weigh at birth on average 250 g less than babies of other mothers. This lower birthweight has nothing to do with prematurity or with differences in maternal stature but is due to intrauterine growth retardation associated with chronic maternal anaemia. Any severe maternal anaemia may result in retardation of intrauterine growth so long as the maternal haemoglobin remains under 10 g/dl and the PCV under 0·30 throughout pregnancy (Harrison and Ibeziako, 1973); this is often the case in Hb-SS, but not in Hb-SC or Hb-S/β^+thal (see Table 7.1).

Antenatal care

General principles and management
Antenatal care should aim at the prevention of severe anaemia and at the early recognition and effective treatment of medical and obstetric complications. In women with sickle-cell disease, antenatal care should begin in the first eight weeks of pregnancy. They should attend the antenatal clinic once a fortnight until the thirtieth week, and thereafter once weekly. At each attendance, careful search must be made for evidence of bacterial infection, painful crises, trauma, and enlargement of the spleen and liver. In addition to measuring the blood pressure, testing the urine for proteins and carrying out the usual palpation of the uterus and its contents, it is absolutely essential to estimate and record the haematocrit or haemoglobin level. Once a complication is found, treatment in hospital will be necessary in every case.

Prevention and treatment of anaemia
For this purpose, all pregnant women with sickle-cell disease must be given tablets of folic acid throughout pregnancy and in the puerperium. Additional requirements include iron in places where iron deficiency is common, and antimalarials in areas where malaria is endemic, for example in West Africa.

Folic acid tablets 5 mg daily are usually effective in the prevention of severe anaemia. However, some women may fail to take this medication at home. For this reason, it is wise to make all women swallow a single dose of folic acid (30 mg) at each visit to the antenatal clinic. Where supplements of iron are needed, ferrous sulphate tablets 200 mg daily will often suffice. As far as malarial chemoprophylaxis is concerned, in West Africa, a most useful regime is to give oral chloroquine 600 mg of base at the first visit to the antenatal clinic, and thereafter pyrimethamine 25 mg once weekly or proguanil 100 mg daily. A regime of one proguanil and one folic acid tablet daily is easy to remember and has a high acceptance by patients, especially those who are regular attenders at the sickle-cell clinic when they are not pregnant.

The above measures are often effective in maintaining the haemoglobin concentration at levels of 6 to 9 g/dl in Hb-SS, and around 10 g/dl or more in both Hb-SC disease and Hb-S/β^+thal. Should the haemoglobin level drop by 1·5 g/dl, or should it be under 6 g/dl in Hb-SS and under 7 g/dl in Hb-SC or Hb-S/β^+thal, treatment in hospital will be required.

The place of blood transfusion
Transfusion will be needed whenever life is threatened by haemorrhage or by severe anaemia and its complications. In deciding whether or not to give blood transfusion, the following factors should be taken into consideration: (i) the severity of anaemia, (ii) the stage pregnancy has reached and (iii) the absence or presence of associated diseases and complications, such as bacterial infections, cardiac failure and painful crises.

Packed red blood cell transfusion. When the haemoglobin level is 5 to 6 g/dl, a slow transfusion of packed blood cells (from one unit of blood of Hb-electrophoretic type AA) daily should be given until the haemoglobin is around 8 g/dl.

If the haemoglobin level is below 5 g/dl, or where heart failure is already present, an intravenous injection of either frusemide 40 mg or ethacrynic acid 50 mg should be administered about 15 minutes before blood transfusion is started. These rapidly acting potent diuretics (but not other diuretic agents) are effective in preventing acute pulmonary oedema (Harrison *et al*, 1971).

Sometimes, anaemic patients with sickle-cell disease are seen for the first time when their pregnancies have already reached 36 weeks of gestation, with the haemoglobin level still less than 8 g/dl. In such cases, it is unlikely that haematinics alone will succeed in raising the haemoglobin to safe levels before the onset of labour. For this reason, the transfusion of packed blood cells will be required.

Exchange blood transfusion. If gross anaemia (Hb < 5 g/dl) is present when delivery or abortion is imminent, direct transfusion of packed blood cells with rapidly acting diuretics will take too long in correcting the anaemia fully before the expulsion of the abortus or delivery of the baby. Should these events take place with the patient still very anaemic, blood loss at the third stage of labour, or at operative delivery or abortion, will almost certainly kill the patient. Exchange blood transfusion gives the best results in such cases, and it also has a place in the treatment of pseudotoxaemia. The technique of exchange transfusion is described fully by Fullerton and Turner (1962). The procedure involves an infusion of about 1200 ml of packed cells from an Hb-AA compatible donor and a concurrent venesection of about 1400 ml, the whole operation taking between 10 and 30 minutes to complete; care must be taken to avoid air embolism.

High transfusion regimes. Apart from the above indications, there is increasing support for the idea that pregnant women with sickle-cell disease need repeated blood transfusions throughout pregnancy in order to maintain the circulating haemoglobin at fairly high levels. The argument is that by keeping the haemoglobin level high, bone marrow activity is depressed, the synthesis of Hb-S is suppressed, and it should therefore be possible to lower the incidence of crises. This line of treatment has not found favour universally because there is no convincing clinical evidence that it is effective in improving the results of pregnancy. Furthermore, repeated transfusions involve considerable effort and expense, they do not prevent crises, febrile reactions may follow and these may induce unwanted uterine contractions. In tropical Africa, up to 12 per cent of blood donors may have HB_sAg in their blood so that there is a high risk of hepatitis following transfusion. Also, any blood transfusion carries the chance of sensitisation against red cell- or other antigens, so increasing the risk of haemolytic disease of the newborn, besides making subsequent transfusions more hazardous.

Management of painful crises and pseudotoxaemia

In the first place, the underlying causes of the painful crises must be searched for. Even if these are not found, all patients with painful crises must receive broad spectrum antibiotics, such as ampicillin. Adequate fluid and calorie intake must be maintained, if necessary by intravenous infusions. Relief of pain is achieved symptomatically by oral codeine or intramascular pethidine. The haematocrit or haemoglobin concentration is estimated at least twice daily and whenever there is a drop exceeding PCV 0·04 or Hb 2 g/dl in any 24-hour period; the anaemia is corrected by transfusion of packed blood cells.

Heparinisation. When painful crises occur during the dangerous period (that is the end of pregnancy, labour and in early puerperium), there is a high risk that fatal bone marrow embolism may also follow. In such cases, mortality is greatly reduced by adding heparin to the treatment of painful crises. The patient's clotting time is estimated prior to treatment. One method of heparinisation is to give, intravenously, an initial dose of heparin 10 000 iu, repeating its administration four- to six-hourly in sufficient dosage (5000 to 15 000 iu) to maintain the clotting time at about thrice the normal value, or about 17 minutes (Lawson, 1967). Severe uterine haemorrhage and wound haematoma, sometimes life-threatening, occur often enough to indicate that the right dosage has not been found. Giving lower doses of heparin by repeated subcutaneous injections is worthy of a trial. Whatever method is used, treatment by heparin should be continued until the painful crises cease. When heparinisation is in progress, labour may supervene. On such occasions, in order to prevent excessive haemorrhage, it is necessary to reverse the effect of heparin by an injection of protamine sulphate (10 ml of 1 per cent solution) when the second stage of labour is imminent or immediately before an operative delivery. Heparinisation should recommence two hours after delivery and it should be continued for at least four days, when the danger of bone marrow embolism no longer exists.

Pseudotoxaemia. Where pseudotoxaemia is already present late in pregnancy, the danger to fetal and maternal life is very grave indeed. Exchange blood transfusion should be given promptly to raise the haemoglobin level quickly. This should be followed immediately afterwards by rapid delivery of the baby, if necessary by Caesarean section. Heparinisation should commence two hours later. This treatment, though aggressive, has been found to be life-saving in these cases.

Obstetric complications

Complications such as abortion, obstetric haemorrhage, preeclampsia and fetal malpresentation are seen not infrequently in pregnant women with sickle-cell disease. With one exception, these complications occur with equal frequency in the presence or absence of sickle-cell disease. The exceptional case is with preeclampsia, which, during labour, occurs more often in women with sickle-cell disease than in others. For such obstetric complications, standard methods of obstetric management give good results. However, in the case of fetal malpresentation, it is wise to avoid correction by version because of the risk of fetal asphyxia associated with this manoeuvre.

Conduct of labour

All patients must be delivered in a hospital with good blood transfusion facilities.

Following adequate antenatal care, the outlook on labour is good in the majority of cases, and there is no need to resort to induction of labour when there are no obstetric indications for it. Elective Caesarean section has no special advantage unless there are other obstetric indications for it, such as fetopelvic disproportion and placenta praevia. Patients should therefore be allowed to go into spontaneous labour, and spontaneous vaginal deliveries under close supervision should be encouraged. However, because of the risks of infection, anaemia and painful crises, additional precautions are necessary. Parenteral antibiotics must be given four- to six-hourly, and anaemia occurring at this period be corrected by direct transfusion of packed blood cells or by exchange transfusion. Intravenous fluid therapy is essential for the prevention of dehydration and acidosis. Unnecessary trauma to the perineum should be avoided in the second stage of labour, and blood loss in the third stage should be reduced to the minimum by the active form of management. Ergometrine 0·5 mg is given intravenously at the crowning of the fetal head; as soon as the baby is born and the uterus is felt to retract, the placenta should be expelled by controlled cord traction. Immediately afterwards, the lower genital tract must be carefully inspected to see whether there are lacerations; tears and episiotomies should be repaired at the same time, care being taken to achieve good haemostasis and so prevent haematoma. Blood loss exceeding 150 ml is replaced by transfusion of whole blood if the haemoglobin concentration is over 7 g/dl or by packed blood cell transfusion whenever the haemoglobin is under 7 g/dl.

Prolonged labour carries the risk of infection and maternal acidosis, both of which may precipitate painful crises. For this reason, although vaginal delivery gives the best results, there should be no hesitation in terminating labour by Caesarean section when delivery has not taken place after 24 hours' labour.

For operative deliveries, the usual types of anaesthesia are all suitable, provided certain basic considerations are observed. Before anaesthesia is induced, severe anaemia must be corrected, if need be by blood transfusion, and the haemoglobin level raised to at least 9 g/dl. During the anaesthesia, the aim is to avoid sickling and this should be achieved by the prevention of hypotension and hypoxia. Throughout the period of anaesthesia, 30–50 per cent oxygen should be given and blood loss be replaced (see Ch. 6).

The puerperium

The use of antibiotics and the frequent estimation of haemoglobin concentration, which began during labour, should be continued for the first four days of the puerperium. Painful crises require heparinisation until the affected organs are no longer tender. Breastfeeding must be encouraged, and all patients must remain in hospital for at least seven days after normal delivery and for much longer following operative deliveries.

Family limitation

The risks of high parity in addition to those associated with sickle-cell disease are likely to be so great that women with sickle-cell disease should as far as possible be discouraged from having more than three viable pregnancies. When contraception is needed, oral contraceptive agents should *not* be used, as they cause thromboembolism; intrauterine contraceptive devices and barrier methods are preferred, but sterilisation may be best.

Sickle-cell trait and other variants

During pregnancy, sickle-cell trait is largely innocuous and may even confer certain advantages in the indigenous population of tropical Africa. For example, pregnant women with Hb-AS show less intense *P. falciparum* parasitisation (unpublished observations) and are less liable to develop severe anaemia than women with Hb-AA. On the other hand, mothers with Hb-AS show a greater increase in the incidence of significant bacteriuria and among them, fetal loss rises sharply when labour is complicated by factors known to cause hypoxia, such as preeclampsia, antepartum haemorrhage and prolonged labour. Rarely, there may be haematuria from renal papillary necrosis (see Ch. 2).

Observations on the few women with Hb-S/HPFH followed during pregnancy suggest that this condition is entirely asymptomatic.

FURTHER READING

Fullerton, W.T. & Turner, A.G. (1962) Exchange transfusion in the treatment of severe anaemia in pregnancy. *Lancet*, i, 75–78.

Harrison, K.A. (1976) Sickle-cell disease in pregnancy. *Tropical Doctor*, 6, 74–80.

Harrison, K.A., Ajabor, L.N. & Lawson, J.B. (1971) Ethacrynic acid and packed-blood-cell-transfusion in the treatment of severe anaemia in pregnancy. *Lancet*, i, 11–14.

Harrison, K.A. & Ibeziako, P.A. (1973) Maternal anaemia and fetal birthweight. *Journal of Obstetrics and Gynaecology of the British Commonwealth*, 70, 798–804.

Hendrickse, J.P. deV., Harrison, K.A., Watson-Williams, E.J., Luzzatto, L. & Ajabor, L.N. (1972a) Pregnancy in homozygous sickle-cell anaemia. *Journal of Obstetrics and Gynaecology of the British Commonwealth*, 79, 396–409.

Hendrickse, J.P. deV., Harrison, K.A., Watson-Williams, E.J., Luzzatto, L. & Ajabor, L.N. (1972b) Pregnancy in abnormal haemoglobins CC, S-thalassaemia, SF, CF, double heterozygotes. *Journal of Obstetrics and Gynaecology of the British Commonwealth*, 76, 410–415.

Lawson, J.B. (1967) Sickle cell disease in pregnancy. In Lawson, J.B. & Stewart, D.B. *Obstetrics and Gynaecology in the Tropics and Developing Countries*, ch. 7. London: Arnold.

Serjeant, G.R., Sommereux, A.M., Stevenson, M., Mason, K. & Serjeant, B.E. (1979) Comparison of sickle-cell- °thalassaemia with homozygous sickle-cell disease. *British Journal of Haematology*, 41, 83–93.

Radiology of sickle-cell disease

Pathological-radiological correlations

The pathology of sickle-cell disease has been discussed in previous chapters. Basic to the radiological changes are the following processes.

1. The increased viscosity, fragility, haemolysis and phagocytosis of sickled erythrocytes lead to anaemia.

2. The anaemia and associated anoxaemia act as physiological stimuli to the bone marrow to increase haematopoiesis.

3. This in turn leads to bone marrow hyperplasia; the consequent volumetric increase in the marrow thins the trabeculae of the spongy bone in the medullary cavity and the inner aspect of the cortices of the involved bones.

4. The mechanical sludging of sickled erythrocytes produces vaso-occlusion in arterioles, venules and capillaries.

5. This leads to infarcts in the affected organ or tissue.

6. Infarction may be the prelude to superadded infection, but both probably coexist.

7. A reparative process (the end result of 3 to 6 above) may be present in different tissues and organ systems, depending on the response typical for that tissue or organ.

Hands and feet

The earliest radiological manifestation of sickle-cell disease is the dactylitis seen in infancy and early childhood, generally between six months and two years of age (see Ch. 5). Radiography of the hands and feet usually reveals the soft-tissue swelling which is obvious clinically as the hand-foot syndrome. The tubular bones of the hands and feet show a characteristic rectangular shape from marrow hyperplasia. The latter thins the trabeculae and cortices. Occasionally, an associated periosteal reaction may be localised to one bone or affect several bones. Osteolytic foci may be seen in the medullary cavity. These changes (Figs. 8.1 and 8.2) are indistinguishable from those of infarction, and hence the non-commital

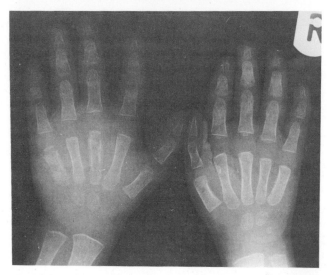

Fig. 8.1 Both hands. Note the generalised thinning of the cortices of the metacarpals and phalanges, which have assumed a rectangular shape as a result of hyperplasia of the bone marrow. Note also the osteolytic foci and periosteal reaction in the shafts of the left third and fifth metacarpals, with the associated soft-tissue swelling.

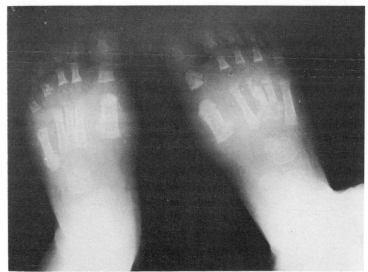

Fig. 8.2 Both feet. Osteolytic foci, infarction and/or osteitis in metatarsals are similar to those seen in the hands (Fig. 8.1). The associated soft-tissue swelling is remarkable.

term *osteitis* is applied in preference to osteomyelitis. Deformities of a digit may occur after healing. These could result in shortening and broadening of the digit. A false appearance of vertical splitting

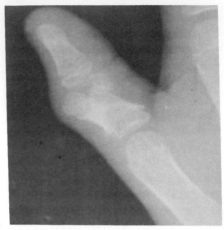

Fig. 8.3 Thumb. Note the end result of an old healed infarct in the proximal phalanx of the thumb. It is shortened, broadened, 'double-headed' and has a conical basal epiphysis.

followed by reunion of the shaft of the affected phalanx, metacarpal or metatarsal may produce a double-headed or 'duplex' digit (Fig. 8.3). Retardation of bone age may occur at the carpal bones. A wedge-shaped epiphysis from an infarct at the central portion of

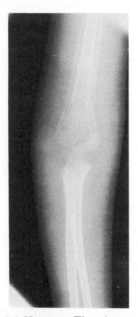
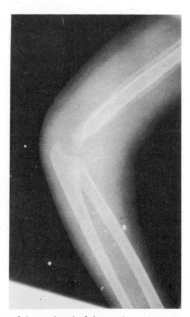

Fig. 8.4 Humerus. There is encasement of the entire shaft by periosteal new bone giving the 'tram-line' appearance. This is one form of the so-called bone-within-bone.

the metaphyseal plate may be seen —— the so-called conical epiphysis (Fig. 8.3) or 'peg-in-hole' deformity. In the adolescent with sickle-cell disease, the tubular bones of the hands and feet may appear unduly elongated —— 'pseudo-Marfan's syndrome sign' (Lagundoye, 1970).

Long bones

The commonest lesion of the long bones is infarction (Figs 8.4 and 8.5). This may affect the entire shaft or may be restricted to the upper, middle or lower thirds, or to subsegments of these areas. The lesions may be multiple, and sometimes bilateral and symmetrical (Fig. 8.5). Such symmetrical bilateral distribution favours the diagnosis of sickle-cell disease rather than some other disorder. Where the metaphyseal plate is involved, this may lead to alteration

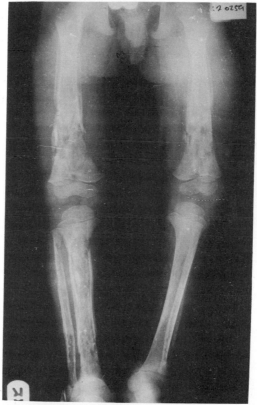

Fig. 8.5 Lower limbs. Note the multiple foci of osteomyelitis symmetrically involving the femora and both fibulae. The entire shaft of the right tibia is also involved. *Salmonella typhi* was the organism cultured from the pus obtained from a discharging sinus in the left thigh.

in shape or to deformity of the epiphysis with consequent disturbance of its growth. A trough-like channel in the medullary cavity
may mark the tract of migration of the densely sclerotic infarcted
portion of the metaphyseal plate away from the unaffected portion
as growth proceeds, and may be seen in adult life long after
epiphyseal closure. Periosteal new bone may appear early and this,
together with osteolytic foci within the spongiosa, makes distinc-
tion between pure infarction and infection (osteomyelitis) difficult
(see Figs 8.1, 8.2, 8.4 and 8.5). In fact, such differentiation is
academic, since both processes probably coexist, the infarction
being the prelude to the infection, and the non-commital term
'osteitis' is preferred. Periosteal or endosteal new bone, or both,

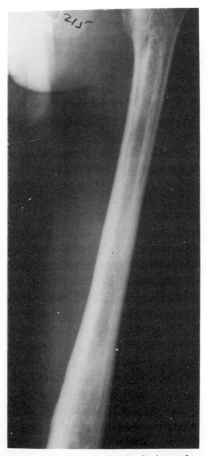

Fig. 8.6 Femur. Note the cortical thickening in the lower femoral shaft and
'bone-within-bone' appearance in the upper part of the shaft; these are the end
results of old healed infarcts.

may appear parallel to the shaft, leading to the so-called tram-line or bone-within-bone appearance. Healed infarcts may leave their marks in the diaphysis: localised medullary sclerosis and rarely 'bone-within-bone' appearance (Fig. 8.6).

The spine

The changes are summarised in Figure 8.7.

1. There may be biconvexity of disc spaces.

2. There may be a trough-like depression of the central portion of the vertebral end plates (at the bottom of which the dense infarcted segment or its remnant may be seen), producing a 'cod-fish vertebra' appearance. Its pathophysiology has been explained by

SPINE INVOLVEMENT IN SICKLE-CELL DISEASE

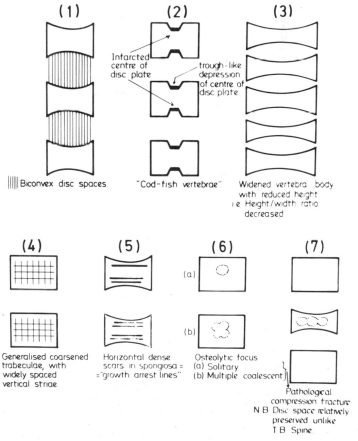

Fig. 8.7 Changes in the vertebral column in sickle-cell disease.

Reynolds (1966) on the basis of the dual blood supply to the vertebral end plate, a view that is analogous to Cockshott's (1963) explanation for the development of the 'peg-in-a-hole' or 'conical epiphysis' at the phalanges.

3. The height-width ratio of the vertebral body may be decreased. The vertebrae appear wider but shorter than normal (see Fig. 8.15) thus mimicking changes seen in Paget's disease or haemangioma of a vertebra; in sickle-cell disease, however, several vertebrae are involved, while in the former two conditions the lesion is usually monostotic.

4. Occasionally, osteolytic foci, which frequently coalesce, may be seen in the spongiosa of the vertebral bodies. Several vertebrae may be involved; the author has seen osteitis involving as many as 10 vertebrae.

5. Collapse or a pathological compression fracture may complicate sickle-cell osteitis of the vertebrae. The differentiation from tuberculosis of the spine can be difficult. In general, the osseous stigmata of sickle-cell disease will be seen in the vertebrae and other bones, while the disc spaces will be relatively well preserved; in contrast, diminution of disc spaces is an early feature of tuberculosis of the spine (Obisesan *et al.*, 1977). The difficulty is further compounded by the wide prevalence of both conditions in Africa.

6. Dense linear horizontal sclerotic scars may be seen in the vertebral spongiosa; they are analogous to the so-called growth-arrest-lines of Harris seen in the long bones in growing children (Lagundoye, 1970).

The skull (Fig. 8.8)
The commonest change is widening of the diploe, most obvious in the frontal and parietal eminences, which are the regions of the bossing of the cranial vault seen clinically (Fig. 8.9). At the base of the skull, the orbital plates of the frontal bone also show a thickened and widened diploe in continuity with that seen in the vertical portion of the frontal bone. A uniform parallelism of the contour of the outer and inner tables over a wide portion of the vault in the lateral radiograph of the skull, especially in the frontal and parietal regions, is often pathognomonic of sickle-cell disease. Curvilinear lamellation within the diploe is a common finding and is due to the trabeculae of its spongy bone running parallel to the curvature of the outer and inner tables (Lagundoye, 1970); this has been confirmed histologically (Williams *et al.* 1975). This curvilinear trabecular pattern or 'onion-peel lamellation' (Fig. 8.10) is far more common than the vertical trabecular arrangement responsible for

SKULL INVOLVEMENT IN SICKLE – CELL DISEASE

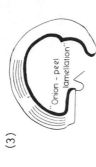

(1)

NOTE: (a) Thinned outer table
(b) Widened diploe, with dense uniform texture extending to orbital roofs (d)
(c) Absolute parallelism of inner and outer tables of vault.

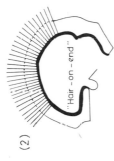

(2)

Intradiploic vertical stripe - like arrangement of trabecular pattern = "hair - on - end" illusion

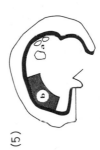

(3)

"Onion - peel lamellation"

Intradiploic curvilinear lamellation of trabecular pattern

(4)

Combination of (2) and (3) in same patient

(5)

Other vault changes
(a) Osteitis
(b) Generalised coarsened diploic texture

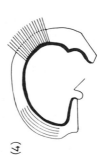

(6)

JAW CHANGES (MANDIBLES)

(a) Prognathus
(b) Coarsened trabeculae of alveolar margin
(c) Well - defined lamina dura

Fig. 8.8 Changes in the skull in sickle-cell disease.

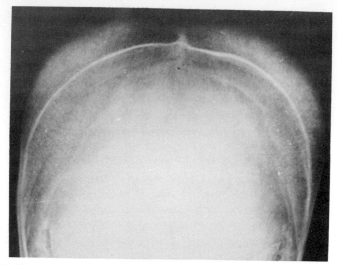

Fig. 8.9 Bossing of the skull. Note the grossly thickened cranial vault, corresponding to clinically overt bossing. The diploic space is wide and filled with spongy bone of uniform texture. Note the indistinctness of the outer table and 'thinning' of the inner table, both a result of hyperplasia of the bone marrow in the dipioe.

the so-called hair-on-end appearance (Fig. 8.11). Osteolytic foci may be seen rarely in the vault.

The alveolar margins of the jaws may show a coarse trabecular pattern with a well-defined cortical bone (lamina dura) for the tooth sockets. A prognathus of the jaw ('gnathopathy') has been described (see Ch. 5 and 6).

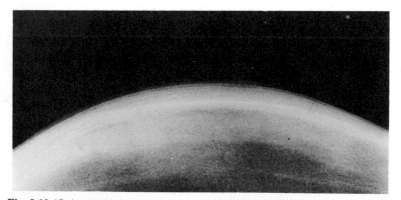

Fig. 8.10 'Onion-peel lamellation' of the cranial vault. The curvilinear arrangement of the intradiploic trabeculae parallel to the curvature of the outer and inner tables of the vault shown here is a more common arrangement than the 'hair-on-end' pattern.

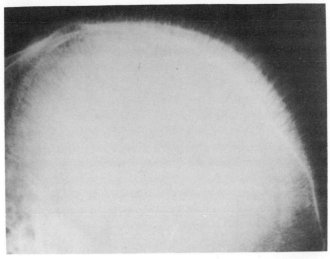

Fig. 8.11 The 'hair-on-end' appearance in the cranial vault. This is an illusion produced by the arrangement of the bony trabeculae within the widened diploe in parallel strips, vertical to the curvature of the inner table.

Flat bones

The scapulae, pelvis and ribs tend to be wider than normal, this being more obvious in the lower ribs. Their trabeculae tend to be arranged in lamellae which run parallel to their curvature (Fig. 8.12). With age, the trabeculae become progressively coarser and eventually a uniform dense sclerosis of the entire ribs may result (see Fig. 8.15), a picture analogous to that seen in myelofibrosis (Lagundoye, 1970).

Joints

The larger joints are prone to aseptic necrosis; the hips, knees, ankles, shoulders and elbows are affected in that order of frequency. Only a portion of the articular surface is involved. In weight-bearing joints, the affected portion of the articular subchondral cortex becomes fragmented and depressed below the articular surface. In the hip, the lesion closely mimics Perthes' disease (Barton and Cockshott, 1962; Obisesan and Bohrer, 1972). In the latter condition, the entire articular surface of the femoral head tends to be involved, while in sickle-cell disease aseptic necrosis is localised to only a fraction of the joint surface (Figs 8.13 and 8.14). Moreover, Perthes' disease tends to present in children aged five to ten years, while aseptic necrosis is seen in adolescent and adult patients with sickle-cell disease. Aseptic necrosis has been said to be more common in Hb-SC than in Hb-SS disease (Diggs, 1967).

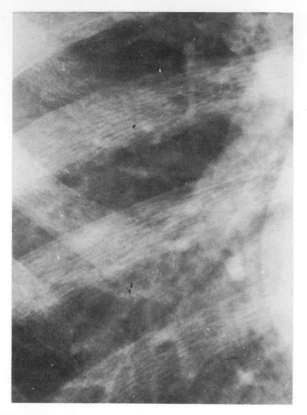

Fig. 8.12 Ribs. Close-up view of the ribs of a patient with sickle-cell anaemia showing the arrangement of the coarse trabeculae of spongy bone in strips that are parallel to the curvature of the long axis of the ribs. The ribs themselves are wider than normal, and their cortices are thinned beyond recognition as a result of hyperplasia of bone marrow from increased haematopoiesis.

Bone marrow

The hyperplasia of the bone marrow exerts pressure on the adjacent trabecula and inner cortex, and results in their thinning, as has been mentioned in connection with changes in the long and short tubular bones as well as in the ribs. Osteolytic foci in the marrow cavity, indicating osteitis or infarct, have been described above. Fat necrosis may resolve by leaving amorphous calcific deposits within the marrow cavity. If the process goes on long enough, the calcification will be replaced by ossification which is another pathway for the production of the 'bone-within-bone' appearance.

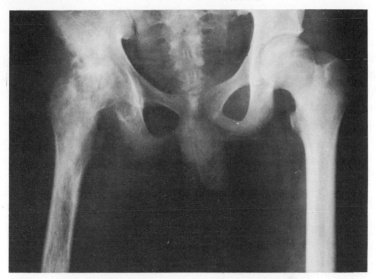

Fig. 8.13 Hips. Note the disuse osteoporosis of the right hip and upper femur. Note the partial collapse of the superolateral segment of the femoral head from the aseptic necrosis (early phase).

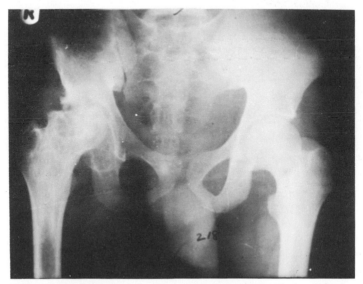

Fig. 8.14 Hips. Same patient as in Figure 8.13 one year later. The involved area is now flattened and more sclerotic and shows fragmentation of the subchondral cortex; there is an associated lipping of the opposing acetabular roof and a degenerative cyst in the widened femoral neck (late phase).

The spleen

The plain film may show splenomegaly in children, and this is not uncommon in areas endemic for malaria. When infarcts occur in the spleen, the associated perisplenitis can produce a left basal, 'sympathetic' pleurisy and an elevated left hemidiaphragm. Splenic infarcts may be followed by colliquative necrosis in the centre of the infarcted area. Splenic abscesses may also develop in the infarcted zone. Mottled gaseous translucencies may be seen in the so-called pyogaseous abscess (Cockshott and Weaver, 1962; Kolawole and Bohrer, 1973). These abscesses can rupture into the peritoneal, pleural or pericardial cavities.

Calcification in the splenic area should raise the suspicion of the possibility of sickle-cell disease being present. Of eleven cases of

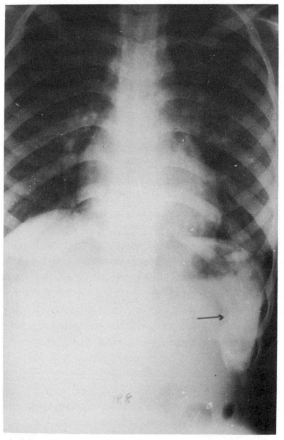

Fig. 8.15 The chest. Note the sclerotic ribs and the dense opacity of the shrunken siderofibrotic spleen (black arrow).

splenic calcification diagnosed at Ibadan, nine were Hb-SS and two were Hb-SC; three of the patients were below 15 years of age, and the rest were adults. The calcifications are of four types (Lagundoye, 1971):

1. curvilinear from old perisplenitis
2. thick amorphous from healed intrasplenic infarcts
3. miliary nodular calcification leading ultimately to the shrunken siderofibrotic spleen, which is in effect an autosplenectomy (Fig. 8.15)
4. uniform parenchymatous opacity.

It should be noted that mixtures of the four types of calcification can occur in various combinations.

The kidney

Intravenous urography (Fig. 8.16) usually shows enlarged kidneys with minimal blunting of the calyces to moderate caliectasis (Plunket *et al.*, 1965; Daini, S.S.A., personal communication). Less commonly, spontaneous haematuria is seen in sickle-cell disease and also sickle-cell trait, resulting from papillary necrosis (Eckert *et al.*, 1974). The changes are similar to those of papillary necrosis following drug abuse. Intravenous urograms on 181 patients with sickle-cell disease showed deformities of calyceal pattern attributable to scars of previous symptomless papillary necrosis (Daini, S.S.A., personal communication).

The gallbladder

Although gallstones are infrequent in Nigerians (see Ch. 6), they are seen in patients with sickle-cell anaemia much more frequently and at a much younger age than in the general population, both in Nigerians (Akinyanju and Ladapo, 1979) and in black Americans (Lachman *et al.*, 1979). In an ongoing study in Ibadan of patients with sickle-cell disease, oral cholecystography tends to show poorer concentration of the contrast in the gallbladder, which implies some element of diminished function when compared with control subjects (Taiwo, A.O., personal communication).

Central nervous system

Neurological disorders associated with sickle-cell disease include disturbance of consciousness, convulsions, meningitis, cranial nerve palsies and cerebrovascular accidents (Adeloye and Odeku, 1970). Cerebral angiography may show vascular displacement, vaso-occlusion of major vessels or evidence of hydrocephalus, as

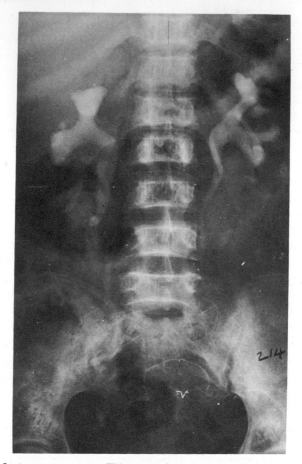

Fig. 8.16 Intravenous urogram. This was performed as part of the investigation for hypertension in a male aged 25 years. There is bilateral clubbing of the calyces and slight dilatation of the ureters. Note the sclerosis of the bones generally, and especially the reduced height and increased width of the vertebral bodies, which also have a coarsened trabecular pattern. There is a slight biconvexity of the lumbar disc spaces. Haemoglobin electrophoresis showed an Hb-SS pattern, thus confirming the radiological suspicion of an haemoglobinopathy.

indicated by excessive bowing of the frontopolar and callosomarginal divisions of the anterior cerebral artery in the lateral arteriogram. The skull changes of sickle-cell disease previously mentioned, when seen in a patient with cerebral symptoms, should increase the suspicion of an intravascular vaso-occlusive phenomenon as a possible causative factor.

The chest
There is often a cardiomegaly with a globular configuration from an

cell disease may quite often arise from X-ray investigations performed in the course of medical examination for diverse reasons, including automobile accidents or other emergencies.

REFERENCES

Adeloye, A. & Odeku, E.L. (1970) The nervous system in sickle-cell disease. *African Journal of Medical Sciences*, **1**, 33–48.

Akinyanju, O. & Ladapo, F. (1979) Cholethiasis and biliary tract disease in sickle-cell disease in Nigerians. *Postgraduate Medical Journal*, **55**, 400–402.

Barton, C.J. & Cockshott, W.P. (1962) Bone changes in hemoglobin SC disease. *American Journal of Roentgenology, Radium Therapy and Nuclear Medicine*, **88**, 523–532.

Cockshott, W.P. (1963) Dactylitis and growth disorders. *British Journal of Radiology*, **36**, 19–26.

Cockshott, W.P. & Weaver, E.J.M. (1962) Primary tropical splenic abscess: a misnomer. *British Journal of Surgery*, **49**, 665–669.

Diggs, L.W. (1967) Bone and joint changes in sickle-cell disease. *Clinical Orthopedics*, **52**, 119–143.

Eckert, D.E., Jonutis, A.J. & Davidson, A.J. (1974) The incidence and manifestations of urographic papillary abnormalities in patients with S hemoglobinopathies. *Radiology*, **113**, 59–63.

Kolawole, T.M. & Bohrer, S.P. (1973) Splenic abscess and the gene for hemoglobin S. *American Journal of Roentgenology, Radium Therapy and Nuclear Medicine*, **119**, 175–189.

Lachman, B.S., Lazerson, J., Starshak, R.J., Vaughters F.M. & Werlin, S.L. (1979) The prevalence of cholelithiasis in sickle cell disease as diagnosed by ultrasound and cholecystography. *Pediatrics*, **64**, 601–603.

Lagundoye, S.B. (1970) Radiological features of sickle-cell anaemia and related haemoglobinopathies in Nigeria. *African Journal of Medical Sciences*, **1**, 315–342.

Lagundoye, S.B. (1971) Splenic calcification in sickle cell disease in Nigerians. *Tropical and Geographical Medicine*, **23**, 135–140.

Obisesan, A.A. & Bohrer, S.P. (1972) Perthes' disease in Nigerians. *Ghana Medical Journal*, **11**, 298–302.

Obisesan, A.A., Lagundoye, S.B. & Lawson, E.A. (1977) Radiological features of tuberculosis of the spine in Ibadan, Nigeria. *African Journal of Medical Sciences*, **6**, 55–67.

Plunket, D.C., Leiken, S.L. & LoPresti, J.M. (1965) Renal radiologic changes in sickle cell anemia. *Pediatrics*, **35**, 955–959.

Reynolds, J. (1966) Re-evaluation of the 'fish vertebra' sign in sickle cell hemoglobinopathy. *American Journal of Roentgenology, Radium Therapy and Nuclear Medicine*, **97**, 693–707.

Williams, A.O. Lagundoye, S.B. & Johnson, C.L. (1975) Lamellation of the diploe in the skulls of patients with sickle cell anaemia. *Archives of Diseases in Childhood*, **50**, 948–952.

early age. This is a result of the hypovolaemic circulation fro
chronic anaemic state. The lungs show multiple interstitial
which cause a generalised loss of translucency to the lung
this, together with coarse trabeculation of the widened rib
Fig. 8.12), gives a characteristic appearance to the chest X-
patients with sickle-cell anaemia. Sclerosis of the ribs and cla
simulating myelofibrosis may be seen in older patients and
sents an end-phase reaction due to the exhaustion of the m
from the compensatory hyperplasia of earlier years.

Abdominal crisis

The plain X-ray of the abdomen during an abdominal crisis
give one of several pictures.

1. It may be normal.
2. There may be non-specific ileus, that is dilatation of b
loops outlined by gas; if this ileus is restricted to the pro
colon as far as the splenic flexure, it indicates a vaso-occlusive
cess in the superior mesenteric artery.
3. There may be multiple fluid levels and distension of
bowel, closely mimicking acute intestinal obstruction. Lac
awareness of this possibility can lead to unwarranted emerge
abdominal surgery, with the attendant risk of general anaesth
initiating a vicious circle of hypoxia, further thromboembolic v
occlusion and infarction in multiple organs and organ systems.
4. There may be no gas or paucity of gas in the bowel loops
5. A sudden increase in splenic shadow may accompany the
called sequestration crisis.

However, none of these changes are specific for abdominal
sis, nor are they always present together in the same patient (Lag
doye, 1970).

SUMMARY

The radiological manifestations of sickle-cell disease are protean.
organ is spared by the disease. Of particular importance are
osseous changes in the long bones, phalanges, metacarpals, m
tarsals, spine, ribs and skull. Curvilinear lamellation of the diplo
the skull is more commonly seen than the 'hair-on-end' app
ance. Splenic abscesses and calcification present characteristic
tures. In sickle-cell abdominal crisis, the clinical and radiolo
changes may be a replica of those seen in acute intestinal obst
tion.

One importance of radiology is that the first suspicion of si

Recent advances and current research in sickle-cell disease

This chapter will attempt to highlight some areas of research in sickle-cell disease where progress which is important and relevant to the theme of this book has been made.

The basis of sickle-cell disease is the sickling phenomenon which occurs when Hb-S is exposed to low oxygen tension. Since theoretically, and in practice, it is easier to analyse this phenomenon than the mechanics of genetic control of synthesis of haemoglobins, it is understandable that, in the last few years, much attention has been focused on investigating the processes involved in sickling, with a view to finding effective therapeutic agents. Significant progress has been made in this direction, and this has given new impetus towards evolving more rational and effective therapeutic measures.

We shall now discuss these areas of progress and subsequently examine therapeutic applications.

Gelation of haemoglobin-S

Gelation of Hb-S is known to precede sickling. *In vitro*, it is one of the easily induced haemoglobin forms, and processes preceding and accompanying gelation have therefore received close attention. For instance, as a necessary precondition to our understanding of Hb-S gelation, it had been necessary (i) to examine the structure of gelled haemoglobin, (ii) to define predisposing conditions for its initiation and development, and (iii) to study its progress to sickling.

The structure of both gelled and sickled haemoglobin has been described in detail using different techniques, including electron and polarising microscopy, and X-ray diffraction. From these observations it was concluded that in states of low oxygen tension, high concentrations of deoxy-Hb-S, such as occurs in the sickled red cell, form tactoids (gels) which appear end-on as ring-shaped stacks arranged in a vertical axis (Dean and Schechter, 1978). Controversy still persists about the exact number of stacks and component pillars or vertical crystals in the tactoids. In recent work, details of contact points as well as of the energy characteristics of the tactoids have been clarified, and it has been shown that in sickle-cell anaemia, one $\beta_s{}^{valine}$ takes part in the intermolecular contact formation and also contributes substantial energy which stabilises the contact point. This would explain in part the observation that at identical haemoglobin concentrations, deoxy-Hb-A does not gel while Hb-S does.

It was also found that, in addition to oxygen tension, oxygen affinity, haemoglobin concentration, 2,3-DPG and pH are some of the factors which affect gelation and sickling. Recent research has resulted in a clearer definition of the ways in which these factors affect the process of gelation and sickling; this has recently been excellently reviewed (Dean and Schechter, 1978). An example of how normal haemoglobins influence the gelation of Hb-S is discussed in some detail below.

The effect of normal haemoglobins on gelation of Hb-S
The study of the amino acid compositon of haemoglobin chains has been useful in helping us understand some aspects of the mechanisms of gelation and sickling. It has been demonstrated that incorporation of new chains into haemoglobin which is already gelled is facilitated if the amino acid sequence of the new haemoglobin chain to be incorporated is similar to that already in the gel. If however, the amino acids or their sequences are different, incorporation of these new chains into the gel either does not occur or is substantially delayed. The gelation of deoxygenated Hb-S is considerably reduced by the addition of normal deoxygenated haemoglobin tetramers of Hb-A or Hb-F. Hb-F is more effective than Hb-A as an inhibitor of gelation of Hb-S. Two possible mechanisms have been suggested. First, Hb-F differs from Hb-S by 20 amino acid residues and is excluded from the gel, whereas Hb-A differs by only one amino acid and some is included. Secondly, in mixtures of two haemoglobins (such as Hb-S + Hb-F or Hb-S + Hb-A), a large proportion of the haemoglobin exists as hybrid tetramers (that is $\alpha_2\beta^S\gamma$ and $\alpha_2\beta^A\beta^S$); thus, Hb-F has a further inhibitory effect on gelation which is dependent on the formation of $\alpha_2\beta^S\gamma$ hybrid tetramers, an action not shared by the $\alpha_2\beta^A\beta^S$ hybrid tetramer (Bookchin *et al.*, 1975).

These findings, together with the high oxygen affinity of Hb-F, may be responsible for the much better clinical features, including physical appearance, noted in patients with sickle-cell anaemia and a high concentration of Hb-F. The observations have generated much interest in the haemoglobin 'switch' mechanism which controls the switch from production of fetal haemoglobin to adult haemoglobin. It is reasoned that if this can be fully understood and mastered, it would be a major breakthrough in the management of sickle-cell disease. Current research activity in recombinant DNA could also provide a useful tool.

The action of ligands

'Ligand' is a chemical term used to describe any atom or molecule which is attached to a central atom — the latter usually a metallic element — in a complex compound. The atoms or molecules used as ligands are almost always expected to be capable of functioning as electron-pair donors in the electron-pair bond formed with the metallic atom. The term is used in the context of this chapter to describe the binding of small molecules, especially oxygen or carbon monoxide, to the iron atom of the haemoglobin molecule. Liganding Hb-S has been observed to delay, if not completely prevent, gelation. The mechanism of action appears to be through competition with normal oxygen binding.

Ligands with methaemoglobins (usually water or OH⁻ ions) have been extensively used in experimental studies, such as changes of volume associated with such binding (Ogunmola *et al.*, 1976). It should, however, be noted that there are important differences in structure and physiological function between methaemoglobin and deoxyhaemoglobin.

The sickled erythrocyte

If Hb-S is withdrawn from the red cell and deoxygenated *in vitro*, it gels. If a concentrated oxygenated Hb-S solution is transferred into an empty normal red cell membrane which is then sealed and deoxygenated, the haemoglobin sickles and the normal membrane assumes the sickle-cell shape. If the experiment is reversed, that is, if oxygenated Hb-A solution is transferred into a red cell membrane of an Hb-SS subject and then deoxygenated, the discoid shape of a normal red cell is retained. This experiment indicates that sickling is an inherent property of Hb-S and not primarily a membrane process.

Irreversibly sickled cells

Sickled cells exist in two forms. In one form, the sickled red cell can revert to normal shape when oxygen tension improves: this is the reversibly sickled cell. In the second form, sickling is irreversible whatever the environmental conditions afterwards. These erythrocytes are called irreversibly sickled cells (ISC). The percentage of ISCs may vary from 5 to 50 per cent in the peripheral blood in some patients during crisis, although the frequency and severity of painful crises do not appear to correlate well with the proportion of ISCs.

Some aspects of function of the sickled cell deserve closer examination. How efficient is such a cell in terms of processes which are essential to its life? It is known that the sickled cell has a partially ineffective K^+, Na^+ and ATP-ase pump. This explains the observation that the sickled red cell leaks Na^+ and K^+, but as this occurs equally in opposite directions, there is no net change in the cell volume. However, with respect to Ca^{2+}, the pump which maintains its cellular distribution is also defective, and this may partially account for the characteristic high intracellular Ca^{2+} observed in the sickled cell. Although these ionic changes have been analysed separately, in practice, the fluxes are balanced and no volume changes occur in the sickled red cell until the sickle/unsickle cycle is repeated a few times. Irreversible changes, including reduction of volume and damage to the membrane, then occur with resultant increased intracellular haemoglobin concentration and sickling.

Reversibly sickled cells are, in some instances, the precursors of ISCs. Similar biochemical changes are observed in the ISCs as in the reversibly sickled cell, except that the disturbances are of a more severe degree in the ISCs. It has also been found that these ISCs retain the sickled shape after all the haemoglobin has been removed, thus showing that permanent damage to the membrane has taken place. The detailed mechanisms of these changes are yet to be fully clarified. It has recently been suggested that the Ca^{2+} changes may be a function of prostaglandin E_2 (PGE_2). It is known that at low oxygen tension PGE_2 causes greater inflow of Ca^{2+} into sickled cells, inducing changes in shape and inhibiting reoxygenation, thereby promoting formation of ISCs (Rabbinowitz and Wolfe, 1977).

One effect of the rigid sickled cell is that it is easily damaged and destroyed. A second effect, which may not be so clear, is that it leads to increased viscosity of blood — the so-called rheological effect. This latter consequence has been demonstrated by measuring filtration rates of deoxygenated normal or Hb-S-containing red cells in appropriate systems. It has been found that under the conditions of the test, sickled erythrocytes show up to 15 times greater resistance to flow in the system than normal red cells.

Prenatal diagnosis
One other area of current research which requires brief mention is prenatal diagnosis of genetic diseases. This development has been

applied to the diagnosis of the haemoglobinopathies (Leonard and Kazazian, 1978), and follows from an earlier observation that nine-week-old human fetuses synthesise small but detectable amounts of adult haemoglobin (Hollenberg *et al.*, 1971). The justification for applying these techniques to sickle-cell disease is that the disease satisfies the usual criteria for applying the procedure, namely:

1. the unacceptable burden of the disease
2. its occurrence and high frequency in a well-defined population
3. availability of adequate screening tests to detect parents at risk of producing affected infants
4. incidence of high risk
5. the fact that at present there is no suitable treatment for the disease.

Two methods are now available for the prenatal diagnosis of sickle-cell anaemia and similar disorders. In the first, fetal blood is obtained by placental aspiration, either directly or under visual control through a fetoscope. By using a variety of techniques, the fetal cells can be concentrated and purified from contaminating maternal cells. The cells are then incubated with a radioactively labelled amino acid, and the globins separated on carboxymethyl cellulose urea columns. In Hb-SS, no normal β chains are synthesised. Instead, radioactive β^s chains are found. The technique of fetal blood sampling requires great skill and is definitely risky to the fetus.

The second method utilises the fact that when a restriction endonuclease, Hpa 1, digests normal DNA, the β-globin gene is found in a fragment 7·6 kilobases (kb) long. In a high proportion of subjects with Hb-S, the β-globin gene is found in a new fragment 13·0 kb long, a finding that is being used to diagnose the condition prenatally (Kan and Dozy, 1978). In this system, DNA is extracted from cells from the amniotic fluid; these are collected by amniocentesis, which is both relatively simple and safe for the infant; but further developments are required before the procedure can be made cheap and readily available.

However, inspite of the great advances which have been made in solving the technical problems, the human problems still loom large. In tropical countries, it is legitimate to ask how justified it would be to devote large fractions of scarce resources to this procedure, particularly as there is no assurance that affected couples would accept the suggestion to terminate the pregnancy should all the tests support a diagnosis of haemoglobinopathy in the fetus. It is known that many a couple who have been offered this option have chosen to carry the pregnancy to term and deliver and care for the affected child rather than agree to terminate the pregnancy.

Bone marrow transplantation

Organ transplantation is an area of active current interest. Bone marrow transplantation has been undertaken as an adjunct to other therapeutic measures, or as a form of treatment itself, in a number of haematological and related disorders, such as aplastic anaemia, haematological malignancies and immunodeficiency disease. Application of this procedure to the management of sickle-cell disease has also received active consideration, the limitations of the procedure notwithstanding.

Therapeutic applications in sickle-cell disease

In the last decade, more than 60 chemotherapeutic agents have been proposed as having specific actions in preventing or curing sickle-cell crises. None of these have been shown to be as effective as had earlier been anticipated. Some have proved to be too toxic (e.g. cyanate and iodoacetate). Others, such as glucocorticoids, have unacceptable risks which make their use inadvisable. In some instances, original claims of antisickling properties have not been confirmed (e.g. piracetam), while others have been shown to be no more effective than placebos in double-blind trials (e.g. urea). The majority have not been submitted to properly conducted double-blind trials.

The outline below indicates some possible sites of action of a drug which prevents or shortens the duration of a sickle-cell crisis.

1. The Hb-S molecule may be altered so as to prevent gelation or increase the delay time of progress from gelation to sickling.

2. The red cell membrane may be changed so as to resist the damage to it caused by sickled haemoglobin.

3. The secondary complication of thrombosis could be prevented by action on platelets and other haemostatic factors. The extent of the involvement of these systems in either initiating or maintaining the sickling process, however, remains to be fully established.

4. The blood flow through tissue, and hence oxygenation of tissue, could be increased by causing vasodilation or by decreasing blood viscosity.

Some of the recently proposed chemotherapeutic agents are listed in Table 9.1. The general physician is strongly recommended *not* to prescribe, at present, any of these agents to patients with

Table 9.1   Some chemotherapeutic agents which have been proposed in the prevention or treatment of sickle-cell crisis. **None of these are recommended for general use.**

Suggested site of action	Therapeutic agent	Comments and references
Haemoglobin-S molecule	Urea	Clinically ineffective (see text) (Co-operative Urea Trials Group, 1974)
	Cyanate	Toxic (May and Huehns, 1974)
	Pyridoxal	No blind trial (Kark *et al.*, 1978)
	Piracetam	Ineffective (Costa *et al..* 1979; Franklin, 1980)
	Aromatic alchohols and acids	See text
	Peptides	See text
	DBA and other *Fagara* derivatives	See text
Red cell membrane	Glucocorticoids	Unacceptable side effects (Bennett and Rosner, 1979)
	Zinc	No blind trial (Brewer *et al.*, 1977)
	Iodocacetate	Toxic (Costa *et al.*, 1979)
	Vincamine	Ineffective (Roth *et al..* 1978)
Antithrombotic	Aspirin-dipyridamole	No blind trial (Chaplin *et al.*, 1980)
Increased blood flow	Hydergine	Inconclusive blind trial (Begue *et al.*, 1978)

sickle-cell disease, as none have been proved effective, and some are toxic. Furthermore, physicians are advised to resist any proposal to prescribe any drug in the prevention or treatment of sickle-cell crisis unless such drugs have been shown to be acceptably free from toxicity, and effective in well-conducted double-blind clinical trials.

Urea. It has already been indicated that much progress has been made in our understanding of the molecular processes involved in gelation and sickling. This understanding has led to the introduction of newer therapeutic proposals, such as the use of urea (Murayama, 1966; Nalbandian *et al.*, 1971; Co-operative Urea Trials Group, 1974) and cyanate (Cerami and Manning, 1971) in the management of sickle-cell crisis. Although the initial euphoria of the 'urea era' has since yielded to realism, this failure has had salutary effects. For example, during the urea era, new methods for detailed analysis of haemoglobin gelling and sickling were developed and some older ones refined. These have subsequently been applied to testing new agents for antigelling and antisickling properties. These improved techniques include sickling assays, minimum gelling concentration assays, determination of haemoglobin solubility, gelation kinetics, oxygen affinity assays, microrheorhologic tests and sickle and red cell/Nasalature interactions.

Although it is now clear that some of these techniques may not have immediate therapeutic applications, they have none the less enabled us to approach investigations of new drugs in a more systematic manner. For instance, examination of potential agents for therapeutic effects and mechanisms of action can be investigated for their destabilising effect on sickling (chaotropic activity), for their effect on delay time of intracellular gelation in relation to capillary transit time (Eaton et al., 1976; Sunshine et al., 1978), or by their stearic or covalent bonding effect on oxygen affinity among others. Carbamoylation agents are, for example, thought to exercise their beneficial effect on Hb-S properties by increasing its affinity for oxygen.

Peptides. Another approach to these studies has been to synthesise peptide chains which resemble the amino terminal portion of the β^S chain. The intention was to interact such peptide portions with the corresponding β^S chain and thus disrupt the β^S stable points of interaction. In effect, these peptide chains would act like other chaotropic agents. Aromatic amino acids and phenylalanine-containing tripeptides and tetrapeptides, which have been investigated for this type of activity, have been shown to increase the solubility of deoxy-Hb-S and inhibit gelation (Votano et al., 1977).

Aromatic alcohols and acids. Another group of agents which have been shown to manifest 'stereospecific' inhibition of gelation and sickling include aromatic alcohols and acids. The functional groups in these agents have been found to be both an aromatic group and a hydrogen-donor group. This is very useful information, as it opens the way for organic chemists to synthesise such agents easily.

Fagara zanthoxyloides. In this connection, the recent development of a synthetic organic compound, 3,4-dihydro-2,2-dimethyl-2H-1-benzopyran-6-butyric acid (DBA), by chemists at Ibadan University (Ekong et al., 1975) deserves mention. This compound was derived from zanthoxyllol, an alcohol-soluble extract from the roots of the plant *Fagara zanthoxyloides lam* (*Zanthoxylum zanthoxyloides watern*) or 'orin ata' in the Yoruba language. These roots are widely used as 'chewing sticks' for cleaning teeth by many Nigerians, especially in the south-western States of the country.

The original observation which had led to these developments was the discovery by Sofowora and colleagues that the aqueous extract of the plant 'manifested both antimicrobial and red cell preserving properties in blood agar plates' (El Said *et al.*, 1971). It was shown subsequently that the crude aqueous extract could also reverse both sickling and crenation in erythrocytes *in vitro* (Sofowora and Isaacs, 1971). Aqueous extracts were found to be non-toxic to experimental animals, and it was claimed from preliminary clinical trials that regular administration to patients with sickle-cell disease reduced the incidence of painful episodes (Isaacs-Sodeye *et al.*, 1975).

These reports prompted a reexamination of some earlier investigations, which had focused attention only on the contents responsible for the spicy taste of the roots of the plant (Eshiet and Taylor, 1966). A result was the isolation, characterisation and synthesis of the compounds zanthoxyllol, fagaramide and fagarol from the roots of the plant (Enyinihi, 1974). Tests on zanthoxyllol suggested that it possessed antisickling properties. The compound was subsequently modified to yield the analogue 3,4-dihydro-2, 2-dimethyl-2H-l-benzopyran-6-butyric acid (DBA), which appeared to be a more potent antisickling agent than zanthoxyllol (Ekong *et al.*, 1975). It inhibits gelation in haemoglobin solutions (Poillon and Bertles, 1977), but it is not clear whether it acts as a stereospecific inhibitor. Its precise site of action in relation to the red cell is also not clear. While some suggest that it can enter the red cell to inhibit sickling (Ekong *et al.*, 1975), others are of the view that it cannot (Honig *et al.*, 1978).

Another agent, 2-hydroxymethylbenzoic acid, obtained from the ether-soluble fraction of the aqueous root extract of the same plant is reported to manifest anti-sickling activity (Sofowora *et al.*, 1975). However, its mode of action has not yet been clarified. Other benzoic acid derivatives of the same roots, such as vanillic acid and p-hydroxybenzoic acid, are also believed to possess antisickling properties (Sofowora *et al.*, 1975). Confirmatory evidence for some of these will doubtless be forthcoming soon.

For now, it needs be said that another Pandora's box appears to have been opened from which, with great care, the patients with sickle-cell disease may obtain some relief. Recent reports of potent procoagulant activity *in vitro* in the crude aqueous extract of *Fagara* (Essien and Okogun, 1976) emphasise the need for caution in the use of such forms of products in the management of sickle-cell disease.

SUMMARY

Different aspects of the progress in our understanding of sickle-cell disease, and of research activities which are considered relevant to the theme of this book, are reviewed. Although much progress has been made in the development of new drugs for the management of sickle-cell thrombotic crisis (this follows naturally from our greater understanding of the mechanisms of Hb-S gelation and sickling), little real success has been achieved.

Other areas of active work which, if successful, could bring a more lasting solution to the problem have been referred to briefly. These include the 'switch' mechanism in haemoglobin synthesis, where current interest in recombinant DNA research could provide a useful tool, and bone marrow transplantation.

The need to examine critically claims of traditional cures is emphasised by developments achieved so far in research into constituents of the *Fagara zanthoxyloides lam* plant, some of which have been shown to possess antisickling properties.

ACKNOWLEDGEMENTS

I am grateful to Drs (Mrs) David-West, Oluboyede and Williams, Consultants in the Department of Haematology, University of Ibadan, for their helpful criticisms and comments. I am also grateful to Professor J.I. Okogun and Dr G.B. Ogunmola of the Department of Chemistry, University of Ibadan, for their helpful criticisms. Professor A.E. Sofowora, Department of Pharmacognosy and Director of the Drug Research Unit, University of Ife, Ile-Ife, kindly sent me some of his publications on *Fagara zanthoxyloides*. Mr O. Oladepo kindly typed the manuscript.

REFERENCES

Begue, P., Bertrand, E., Bonhomme, J., David, M., Coullet, Y., Pierredon, M. & Sankale, M. (1978) Action de la dihydroergotoxine sur la crise drépanocytaire. *Nouvelle Presse Médicale*, 7, 2449–2452.
Bennett, A.J. & Rosner, F. (1979) Glucocorticoid therapy of sickle-cell disease. *Lancet*, ii, 474.
Bookchin, R.M., Nagel, R.L. & Balazs, T. (1975) Role of hybrid tetramer formation in gelation of haemoglobin S. *Nature*, 256, 667–668.
Brewer, G.J., Brewer, L.F. & Prasad, A.S. (1977) Suppression of irreversibly sickled erythrocytes by zinc therapy in sickle cell anemia. *Journal of Laboratory and Clinical Medicine*, 90, 549–554.
Cerami, A. & Manning, J.M. (1971) Potassium cyanate as an inhibitor of the sickling of erythrocytes in vitro. *Proceedings of the National Academy of Sciences USA*, 68, 1180–1183.
Chaplin, H., Alkjaersig, N., Fletcher, A.P., Michael, J.M. & Joist, J.H. (1980) Aspirin-dipyridamole prophylaxis of sickle cell disease pain crises. *Journal of Laboratory and Clinical Medicine* (in press).
Co-operative Urea Trials Group (1974) Treatment of sickle-cell crisis with urea in invert sugar: a controlled trial. *Journal of the American Medical Association*, 228, 1125–1128.
Costa, F.F., Zago, M.A. & Bottura, C. (1979) Effects of piracetam and

iodoacetamide on erythrocyte sickling. *Lancet*, **ii**, 1302.

Dean, J. & Schechter, A.N. (1978) Sickle-cell anemia: molecular and cellular bases of therapeutic approaches. *New England Journal of Medicine*, **299**, 752–763.

Eaton, W.A., Hofrichter, J. & Ross, P.D. (1976) Delay time of gelation: a possible determinant of clinical severity in sickle cell disease. *Blood*, **47**, 621–627.

Ekong, D.E.U., Okogun, J.I., Enyinihi, V.U., Balogh-Nair, V., Nakanishi, K. & Natta, C. (1975) New antisickling agent 3,4-dihydro-2, 2-dimethyl-2H-1 benzopyran-6-butyric acid. *Nature*, **258**, 743–746.

El-Said, F., Fadulu, S.O., Kuye, J.O. & Sofowora, E.A. (1971) Native cures in Nigeria. II. The antimicrobial properties of the buffered extracts of chewing sticks. *Lloydia*, **34**, 172–174.

Enyinihi, V.U. (1974) Synthesis and ultraviolet spectra of 4-substituted coumarins chemistry of the roots of *Fagara zanthoxyloides lam. PhD Thesis*, University of Ibadan.

Eshiet, I.I. & Taylor, D.A.H. (1966) Extractives from *Fagara zanthoxyloides*. *Chemical Communications*, **14**, 467–468.

Essien, E.M. & Okogun, J.I. (1976) Effect of the root extract of *Fagara zanthoxyloides* on blood coagulation. *Thrombosis and Haemostasis*, **36**, 525–531.

Franklin, I.M. (1980) Piracetam and sickle-cell disease. *Lancet*, **i**, 767–768.

Hollenberg, M.D., Kaback, M.M. & Kazazian, H.H. (1971) Adult hemoglobin synthesis by reticulocytes form the human fetus at midtrimester. *Science*, **174**, 698–702.

Honig, G.R., Vida, L.N. & Ferenc, C. (1978) Effects *in vitro* of the proposed antisickling agent DBA. *Nature*, **272**, 833–834.

Isaacs-Sodeye, W.A., Sofowora, E.A., Williams, A.O., Marquis, V.O., Adekunle, A.A. & Anderson, C.O. (1975) Extract of *Fagara zanthoxyloides* root in sickle cell anaemia. Toxicology & preliminary clinical trials. *Acta Haematologica*, **53**, 158–184.

Kan, Y.W. & Dozy, A.M. (1978) Antenatal diagnosis of sickle-cell anaemia by D.N.A. analysis of amniotic-fluid cells. *Lancet*, **ii**, 910–912.

Kark, J.A. Kale, M.P. Tarassoff, P.G. Woods, M. & Lessin, L.S. (1978) Inhibition of erythrocyte sickling in vitro by pyridoxal. *Journal of Clinical Investigation*, **62**, 888–991.

Leonard, C.O. & Kazazian, H.H. (1978) Prenatal diagnosis of hemoglobinapathies. *Pediatric Clinics of North America*, **25**, 631–642.

May, A. & Huehns, E. (1974) Treatment of sickle-cell disease. *Transactions of the Royal Society of Tropicl Medicine and Hygiene*, **68**, 85–91.

Murayama, M. (1966) Molecular mechanism of red cell 'sickling'. *Science*, **153**, 145–149.

Nalbandian, R.M. Schultz, G. Lusher, J.M. Anderson, J.W. & Henry, R.L. (1971) Sickle-cell crisis terminated by intravenous urea in sugar solution — a preliminary report. *American Journal of Medical Sciences*, **261**, 309–324.

Ogunmola, G.B. Kauzmann, W. & Zipp, A. (1976) Volume changes in the binding of ligands to methemoglobin and metmyoglobin. *Proceedings of the National Academy of Sciences*, *USA*, **74**, 4271–4273.

Poillon, W.N. & Bertles, J.F. (1977) Effects of ethanol and 3,4,-dihydro-2, 2-dimethyl-2H-1-benzopyran-6-butyric acid on the solubility of sickle hemoglobin. *Biochemical Biophysical Research Communications*. **75**, 636–642.

Rabbinowitz, I.N. & Wolfe, P.L. (1977) Prostaglandins and erythrocyte sickling. In Silver, M.J., Bryan Smith, J. & Kocsis, J.J. *Prostaglandins in Hematology*, pp. 203–207. New York: Spectrum Publications.

Roth, E., Elbaum, D., Godoy, E. & Nagel, R.L. (1978) Hydergine and vincamine derivative LD 4298 exhibit no anti-sickling properties in vitro. *Nouvelle Revue Française d'Hématologie*, **20**, 644–649.

Sofowora, E.A. & Isaacs, W.A. (1971) Reversal of sickling and crenation in erythrocytes by the root extract of *Fagara zanthoxyloides*. *Lloydia*, **34**, 383–385.

Sofowora, E.A. Isaacs-Sodeye, W.A. & Ogunkoya, L.O. (1975) Isolation and characterisation of an antisickling agent from *Fagara zanthoxyloides* root. *Lloydia*, **38**, 169–171.

Sunshine, H.R., Hofrichter, J. & Eaton, W.A. (1978) Requirements for therapeutic inhibition of sickle haemoglobin gelation. *Nature*, **275**, 238–240.

Votano, J.R., Gorecki, M. & Rich, A (1977) Sickle hemoglobin aggregation: a new class of inhibitors. *Science*, **196**, 1216–1219.

FURTHER READING

Dinterfass, L. (1976) *Rheology of Blood in Diagnostic and Preventive Medicine*, Ch. 6, pp. 203–212. London: Butterworths.

Hercules, J.I., Schechter, A.N., Eaton, W.A. & Jackson, R.E. (eds.) (1974) *Proceedings of the First National Symposium on Sickle Cell Disease*. Bethesda: National Institutes of Health.

Huehns, E.R. (1974) The structure and function of haemoglobin: clinical disorders due to abnormal haemoglobin structure. In Hardisty, R.M. & Weatherall, D.J. *Blood and its Disorders*, Ch. 12. Oxford: Blackwell.

Murayama, M. & Nalbandian, R.M. (1973) *Sickle Cell Hemoglobin: Molecule to Man*. Boston: Little, Brown and Co.

Nalbandian, R.M. (ed.) (1971) *Molecular Aspects of Sickle Cell Hemoglobin. Clinical Applications*. Springfield: Thomas.

Rosa, J. Beuzard, Y. & Hercules, J. (eds) (1979) *Development of Therapeutic Agents for Sickle Cell Disease* Amsterdam: Elsevier/North-Holland Biomedical Press.

APPENDIX I

Routine cellulose acetate electrophoresis for separation of haemoglobins

Equipment
1. Electrophoresis chamber (e.g. Shandon) and power supply
2. DC power pack (e.g. Shandon Vokam)
3. Shandon multi-applicator plate
4. Shandon multi-applicator
5. Filter paper — Whatman No. 1 (46 × 57 cm)
6. Cellulose acetate strips (e.g. Shandon Celagram II)
7. Two kidney dishes (large size)
8. Pasteur pipettes (long type)

Reagents
Analar grade reagents are used throughout.
1. *Buffer*: Tris-EDTA-borate (TEB) buffer, pH 8·9

Tris (hydroxymethyl) amino methane	14·5 g
Ethylenediaminetetracetic acid (EDTA)	1·5 g
Boric acid	0·9 g
Distilled H_2O	to 1 litre

2. *Stock solutions*

(a) Potassium cyanide (KCN)	12·5 g
Distilled water	to 250 ml
(b) EDTA	70 g
Distilled water	to 50 ml

3. *Working solution*

KCN stock solution	2·0 ml
EDTA stock solution	0·3 ml
Distilled H_2O	to 120 ml

4. *Ponceau-S stain*

Ponceau-S	0·2 g
Trichloroacetic acid (TCA)	5·0 g
Distilled H_2O	to 100 ml

5. *Rinsing solution (5 per cent glacial acetic acid)*

Concentrated glacial acetic acid	5 ml
Distilled H_2O	to 100 ml

Procedure

Preparation of electrophoresis chamber and cellulose acetate strips

1. Fix two pieces of filter paper of appropriate size across each shoulder and into each outer compartment of electrophoresis chamber.

2. Pour 100 ml of TEB buffer into each outer compartment and 50 ml into each inner compartment of the chamber.

3. Pour 50 ml of TEB buffer into a large kidney dish.

4. Immerse and leave a cellulose acetate strip (about 17 cm long) in buffer in the kidney dish for at least 10 minutes, but preferably for 15 to 20 minutes.

Preparation of haemolysate

1. Set up a row of 16 small (2·5 ml) glass or plastic tubes.

2. Pipette 0·5 ml working solution into each tube.

3. Using a long Pasteur pipette, add one drop of whole blood from each sequestrene (EDTA) anticoagulated blood sample, remembering to rinse the pipette thoroughly with distilled water between samples. In severely anaemic patients, centrifuge 1 ml of the sequestrene blood specimen, and remove plasma with a Pasteur pipette until the PCV is approximately 0·33 (33 per cent); resuspend these packed cells by shaking, and use one drop of this suspension instead of the original whole blood.

4. Mix the contents of each tube by moderately vigorous tapping of the base of each tube so as to lyse the red cells.

Application of haemolysates to Shandon multi-applicator plate

1. The applicator plate should be placed flat on a smooth surface of the laboratory bench.

2. Using a long Pasteur pipette, apply an extremely small amount (less than half a drop) of each haemolysate sample to each of the 16 segments on the plate. It is helpful if a known control Hb-AA sample is applied to segment 1 and a known control Hb-AS sample to segment 16.

3. With blunt forceps, remove the wet cellulose acetate strip from the kidney dish in which it had been immersed in buffer and remove excess buffer by blotting the strip between two pieces of filter paper.

4. Lay the cellulose acetate strip absolutely flat on a smooth piece of cardboard.

5. Apply the teeth of the Shandon multi-applicator to the haemolysates on the respective segments of the applicator plate.

6. Place the teeth of the multi-applicator on the buffer-impregnated cellulose acetate strip along a line 1.5 cm from one of the lateral margins of the strip. This manoeuvre should be gentle but firm.

Electrophoresis 'run'

1. Remove excess buffer from the parts of the filter paper lying on the shoulders of the electrophoresis chamber using any absorbent material, e.g. tissue paper.

2. Fix the cellulose acetate strip containing the haemolysate samples on both shoulders of the chamber so that samples 1 to 16 are aligned parallel with the shoulders. Hold the strip in position with supports provided so that it covers the inner chamber and rests on both shoulders.

3. Cover the chamber, make the appropriate electrical connections, switch on the DC power-pack and carry out the electrophoresis from cathode to anode at 250 volts (5 to 10 mA) for 15 to 30 minutes. At the end of this period, good separation of the haemoglobins should be obtained.

Staining

1. After the electrophoresis 'run', stain the cellulose acetate strip in a small volume of Ponceau-S stain in a large kidney dish for 5 to 10 minutes. Rinse the stained strip in 5 per cent glacial acetic until excess stain is removed (this usually involves one or two rinses).

2. Remove excess fluid by blotting the strip between two pieces of filter paper.

3. Dry the strip face downwards.

4. Mount the dry stained cellulose acetate strip on a stiff card of appropriate size so as to obtain a permanent record.

Hints for a good result

1. Leave freshly prepared buffer to 'mature' for about four days (shaking vigorously each day) before use in electrophoresis chamber.

2. The longer the buffer in the electrophoresis chamber has been in use, the longer will be the electrophoresis 'run' for a good separation. Usually the 'runs' take about 30 minutes for a good separation when the buffer has been in use for two to three weeks, after which the buffer should be discarded.

3. During a 'run', check the current periodically.

4. A large amount (such as a whole drop) of haemolysate on the segments of the applicator plate results in poor separation. The

best results are obtained when about a third of a drop of haemolysate is placed on each segment.

5. The cellulose acetate strip should be submerged completely in the Ponceau-S stain during staining.

REFERENCE

Lehmann, H. & Huntsman, R.G. (1975) Laboratory detection of haemoglobinopathies. *Association of Clinical Pathologists: Broadsheet 33* (obtainable from the Publishing Manager, Journal of Clinical Pathology, BMA House, Tavistock Square, London, WC1H 9JR, United Kingdom).

APPENDIX II

Solubility test for haemoglobin-S

The test depends on the low solubility of Hb-S in the reduced state. In the method, Hb-S forms a turbid suspension which can flocculate when centrifuged or when left standing overnight.

Reagents

1. *Stock buffer*

Anhydrous potassium dihydrogen phosphate	33·78 g
Anhydrous dipotassium hydrogen phosphate	59·33 g
White saponin	2·50 g
Distilled water	to 250 ml

The stock buffer should be stored at 4°C.

2. *Working solution*. This must be prepared *fresh* immediately before performing the test.

Sodium metabisulphite	100 mg
Stock buffer	10 ml

This is sufficient for 10 tests. Alternatively, so as to save reagents if less than 10 tests are to be performed at any time, 10 mg quantities of sodium metabisulphite may be dispensed into many sealed 8 × 75 mm tubes, each marked to show the level of 1 ml. Stock buffer is added to the mark shortly before use.

Method

Blood may be collected by finger or heel prick, or by venepuncture and added to an EDTA anticoagulated container if other tests are to be performed. One drop (about 0·02 ml) of blood is added to 1 ml of the working solution in a 8 × 75 mm tube and mixed thoroughly. The tube is then centrifuged at 3000 r/min (MSE minor centrifuge setting 9) for five minutes. The tube is removed gently, so as not to disturb the flocculation of precipitated haemoglobin, and examined.

Blood of known Hb-AA, Hb-AS and Hb-SS (if available) is tested at the same time as the unknown sample so as to provide controls for comparison.

Interpretation

Hb-S is precipitated as a sharply defined opaque red band on the surface of the test solution. All other haemoglobins remain in solution.

Normal (Hb-AA) blood. All the haemoglobin remains in solution with the pink to mauve colour of reduced haemoglobin.

Sickle-cell trait (Hb-AS). There is a band of precipitated Hb-S on the surface, and the solution also shows a pink to mauve colour of reduced Hb-A in solution.

Sickle-cell anaemia (Hb-SS). All the haemoglobin is precipitated on the surface, and the solution has a clear straw colour. If Hb-F is in high concentration, for example in infancy, the solution will have a pink mauve colour and the test may be interpreted incorrectly as Hb-AS; the blood film, however, should show the typical Hb-SS picture.

Sickle-cell-haemoglobin C disease (Hb-SC). The solubility test result resembles that of Hb-AS, but the blood film should show target cells and 'pseudo sickle cells'.

Sickle-cell β -thalassaemia. The solubility test result in Hb-S/ β^+thal resembles that of Hb-AS, but the density of the colour of reduced Hb-A in solution tends to be less and the blood film is abnormal. In Hb-S/β°thal, the solubility test resembles Hb-SS.

REFERENCE

Serjeant, B.E. & Serjeant, G.R. (1972) A whole blood solubility centrifugation test for sickle cell hemoglobin: a clinical trial. *American Journal of Clinical Pathology*, **58**, 11–13.

APPENDIX III

A pamphlet for parents and patients with sickle cell disease

SICKLE-CELL ANAEMIA

What is 'anaemia'?
The red substance in the blood is called 'haemoglobin'. When we breathe air into our lungs, haemoglobin carries the important part of the air from the lungs to all over the body. If there is not enough haemoglobin, the person feels short of breath and quickly becomes tired. This is called 'anaemia'.

What is 'sickle-cell anaemia'?
The haemoglobin in the blood is in millions of very small envelopes, called cells. These cells are normally like discs. In some people, the haemoglobin is different and is very sticky. This pulls the blood cells into a shape like that of a curved knife used for cutting grass, called in English a 'sickle'. The sickle cells do not live long in the body, and this weakness of the blood is called 'sickle-cell anaemia'.

Why do some people have sickle-cell anaemia?
Sickle-cell anaemia is given to a child, half from his mother and half from his father. A person who is born with sickle-cell anaemia has it all his life. A person who does not have sickle-cell anaemia will never catch it.

How is sickle-cell anaemia passed from the mother and father to the child?
A man or a woman may have half their blood sickle (S) and half normal (A). This is called 'sickle-cell trait', and may be written AS. When a person is AS half his or her seed carries A and half carries S. If two people with AS marry, this is what can happen:

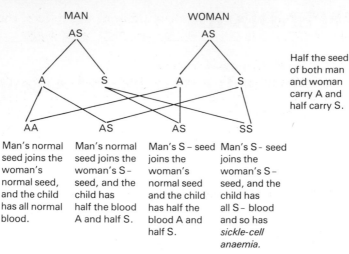

MAN — AS

WOMAN — AS

Half the seed of both man and woman carry A and half carry S.

| Man's normal seed joins the woman's normal seed, and the child has all normal blood. | Man's normal seed joins the woman's S – seed, and the child has half the blood A and half S. | Man's S – seed joins the woman's normal seed and the child has half the blood A and half S. | Man's S – seed joins the woman's S – seed, and the child has all S – blood and so has *sickle-cell anaemia.* |

How common is sickle-cell anaemia?

About one person in five in Nigeria has sickle-cell trait (AS or half sickle blood). This means that one in 25 marriages will be between two people with AS. It will be seen that from their marriages, it is likely that one child in four will have sickle-cell anaemia. That means that about one child in 100 in Nigeria has sickle-cell anaemia.

How does sickle-cell anaemia show?

The blood is weak, which will make the person breathless and easily tired. The blood does not live long in the body. Sometimes, a lot of the blood may be destroyed at once and the person has yellow eyes and dark urine. The sickle-blood cells are destroyed in the liver, which is large, making the belly swollen.

Blood is formed inside the bones in the bone marrow. The bone marrow tries to make more blood to make up the blood destroyed in sickle-cell anaemia. The marrow grows larger in sickle-cell anaemia, making the bones at the back of the skull, the forehead and the upper jaw swell.

Besides there being not enough blood, the sticky sickle cells may clot inside the body. This happens especially in the bones of the hands, arms, feet and legs. There is severe pain and swelling, and the patient has fever. The pain lasts a few days, but sometimes the growth of the bones in children is stopped, and when this happens, the fingers and toes or the whole body may be short. Very occasionally, the bones may be infected, and pus is formed.

The blood may clot in other places, causing nose bleeds, cough, stomach ache, red urine or pain in other parts of the body.

Does sickle-cell trait cause trouble?
Having half haemoglobin S and half haemoglobin A gives almost no trouble and people with sickle-cell trait lead normal lives. In fact, sickle-cell trait is a good thing to have, as a child with AS does not have malaria as badly as a child with all normal haemoglobin.

Can sickle-cell anaemia be cured?
No. A child born with sickle-cell anaemia will have it all his life, but there are many things which can be done to make him strong.

How can we keep a sickle-cell patient well?
Infections very often start the blood cells sickling and sticking together, so making the anaemia worse and causing severe pain. This is called 'crisis'. The commonest infection to start crisis in Africa is malaria. If a sickle-cell person is protected against malaria, he will have far fewer painful crisis attacks, less anaemia and less fever. For this reason every one with sickle-cell anaemia should take regularly medicine which protects him from malaria.

Every patient with sickle-cell anaemia should take also folic acid tablets, which help to make blood.

Other blood tonics and medicines are unlikely to do good, but are more likely to do harm. Do not spend money on iron-containing medicines, as sickle-cell patients do not want iron.

If there is bad fever or illness, the sickle-cell patient should go to see a doctor as soon as possible.

Cold can start crisis. Sickle-cell patients should be kept warm, especially on cold nights, when pyjamas with sleeves and trousers covering to the ankles should be worn. Care should be taken to keep dry and warm in the rainy season, and wet clothes should be changed for dry quickly.

How is painful crisis treated?
When a patient has a small pain crisis he should take aspirin and go to bed. He should keep warm and drink a lot of water. Soluble aspirin (Disprin) is a little better than ordinary aspirin, if it is available.

If the pain and fever are very bad, the patient should go to hospital, where stronger medicine to stop pain can be given.

Many other medicines have been said to shorten the crisis, but at this time, there is no medicine which is proved to help except the drugs which act against pain itself.

How big a handicap is sickle-cell anaemia?

Today, if sickle-cell anaemia is discovered early, care is taken, and the medicines are taken regularly, children with sickle-cell anaemia should grow up to be strong adults with only occasional bone pains. This is true now of children of wealthy families and people who live near the modern hospitals. On the other hand, many children are born of poor parents having bad food and living in villages far away from medical help. They are very weak with anaemia, have frequent fevers and pains. These children are most likely to die young. Most patients with sickle-cell anaemia are somewhere between the lucky ones who have good care always and the unlucky ones who have no treatment.

What happens when a woman with sickle-cell anaemia becomes pregnant?

A woman's resistance to malaria is less during pregnancy, and she will have more fever and more bone pain crisis if she has sickle-cell anaemia. Also, she will need more folic acid when she is pregnant.

A sickle-cell woman who is pregnant must go to a doctor as soon as she knows she is pregnant. It is more important than ever that she receives folic acid and medicine to stop malaria. If she does not have these medicines, she may have severe anaemia, bad bone pains, fever, miscarriage or a small baby born too early.

How can sickle-cell anaemia be prevented?

Sickle-cell anaemia can only happen when both the mother and father have sickle-cell trait or sickle-cell anaemia. A man and a woman who wish to marry can have blood tests done. If they both have sickle-cell trait (AS), they will know that every child they have will have a one in four chance of being born with sickle-cell anaemia.

If man and wife have had a sickle-cell child already, every child they have later still has a one in four chance of having sickle-cell anaemia.

These are the facts. It is for the man and woman to decide whether they shall marry and have children.

What is haemoglobin C?

Haemoglobin C is another abnormal haemoglobin found in about one in twenty people in western and mid-western Nigeria. It is not so bad as haemoglobin S.

Some people will be given S by one parent and C by the other parent. They have then haemoglobin SC. This is a milder form of sickle-cell disease, but it can cause trouble in pregnancy.

If someone is given C by both parents (haemoglobin CC), he has a moderate anaemia, but no painful crisis.

Conclusion

Sickle-patients and parents of sickle-cell patients, REMEMBER:

1. ANTIMALARIAL MEDICINE MUST BE TAKEN REGULARLY
2. FOLIC ACID MUST BE TAKEN EVERY DAY
3. COLD MUST BE AVOIDED
4. SICKNESS OR FEVER MUST BE REPORTED TO THE DOCTOR
5. TAKE CARE, AND LIFE WILL BE LONG AND HEALTH GOOD.

Issued by the Sickle-Cell Club of Nigeria.
Versions in Yoruba, Ibo and Hausa languages are available.

Index

DATE D

JA 31 '97

JAN 19 1998

FEB 2 0 2000

DEC 0 8 2000

JAN 2 5 2002

OCT 2 4 2002

NOV 2 0 2008

Demco, Inc. 38-293